Nutrition and the Later Years

Ruth B. Weg

This monograph is published by the
Ethel Percy Andrus Gerontology Center
University of Southern California

RICHARD H. DAVIS, Ph.D.
Director of Publications and Media Projects

THE ETHEL PERCY ANDRUS GERONTOLOGY CENTER
© 1978

First Printing 1977
Second Printing 1979

THE UNIVERSITY OF SOUTHERN CALIFORNIA PRESS

ISBN 0-88474-042-0

Library of Congress Catalog Card Number 77-91696

Managing Editor: Richard Bohen
Cover Artist:'   Jesus Perez

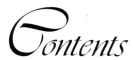

Contents

Preface   i

1. Introduction   1
    The Older Person   1
    Nutrition   9

2. Changing Requirements 17
    Energy Expenditure/Energy Requirements 17
    Adequacy of Dietary Calories 18
    Proteins 19
    Regulatory Nutrients, Low Calorie Intake
        and RDA's 20
    Food/Drug Interactions 22
    Stress/Nutritional Status/Illness 28

3. Nutritional Adequacy 30
    Incidence of Overweight and Obesity 30
    Weight Control: Diet Therapy; Drugs;
        Behavior Modification 33
    Meal Spacing/Nutrition 35
    Low-Calorie Foods; Potential for
        Non-standard Foods 36
    Malnutrition/Undernutrition 37
    Regulatory Substances/General 39
    Major Minerals 41
    Trace Elements: Fe, Zn, Se, Ch 45
    Vitamins: Deficiencies and Functions 48
    Fat-Soluble Vitamins 48
    Water-Soluble Vitamins 51
    Summary 59
    Other Regulatory Substances (water - fiber) . . . 60

4. Functional Changes: Digestive, Metabolic 65
   Gastrointestinal Changes 65
   Digestive Capacity 66
   Protein, Amino Acid Metabolism 69
   Lipid Metabolism 73

5. Pathologies/Diet 77
   Atherosclerosis, Cardiovascular Disease 78
   Cancer, Diet and the Alimentary Tract 84
   Cancer and Nutritional Deficiency 86
   Diverticulosis/Diverticulitis 88
   Diabetes 89
   Conclusions/(Diabetes) 94
   Nutritional Anemias 95
   Osteoporosis 97

6. Behavioral Changes 102
   Taste Capacity/Food Intake 102
   General Attitudes, Beliefs, Practices 103

7. Theories of Aging 111

8. Summation 122
   Summary 122
   Research Priorities 127
   Conclusion 132

Appendix 1 — Glossary 136

Appendix 2 — Dietary 145
           References Cited 162

Appendix 3 — Charts, Figures 200

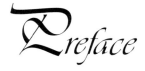

Preface

The demand for information on nutrition and age accelerates for a variety of reasons: in a general way as a response to the increased awareness related to physical fitness; in particular, to the significant increase in the numbers of older persons, more specifically in response to the multiplication of programs for and with older persons; as public acknowledgement and recognition of the older American grow and as the academic area of gerontology widens and deepens its impact across the country.

It would be pleasing to be able to report that all the nutritional and aging facts are 'in', that no more needs to be investigated and understood; that this monograph is a relatively final picture. However — the reality is the lack of enough knowledge related to nutrition as a science, and especially to nutrition and age; the reality is some confusion and honest differences of opinion which require resolution; the reality is the resurgence of interest in nutrition and the potential for food in health maintenance and prevention of illness. There is no simple answer to the pressing concerns about food and aging. Hopefully, this monograph will present the significant data relevant to nutrition in the later years, will identify urgent questions which remain to research and will suggest what current information can be applied to the benefit of the older person today.

I have found this inquiry and my evaluation/interpretation an exciting, timely challenge. One of the attractive features of such a study and its dissemination is the possibility that the quality of dietary intervention would be questioned and improved by the appropriate health professionals and older persons themselves. It is my hope that not only the aged — but the middle aged and all allied health professionals will identify adequate nutrition as a priority. Only in this way can maximum advantage (with minimum disadvantage) of food to the total health of persons in the later years be realized.

My thanks to General Food Corporation for their initial stimulus and support to a critical review of the literature. My appreciation to a number of students, faculty and staff of the Andrus Gerontology Center who helped make this monograph possible. Particular thanks must go to Mrs. Anne Bailey, M.S. nutritionist for her editorial assistance and invaluable advice.

Ruth B. Weg, Ph.D.
Andrus Gerontology Center

"Knowledge, that tendeth but to satisfaction is but as a courtesan, which is for pleasure and not for fruit or generation . . . the sure and lawful goal of the sciences is none other than this: that human life be endowed with new discoveries and power . . .

Francis Bacon — 17th Cent.

Introduction   *1*

THE OLDER PERSON

HOW MANY, HOW OLD

The older person in America is increasing in number at a faster rate than the under 65. This fact is reflected in the change in the median age from 27.9 years in 1970 to 28.8 in 1975, 29.0 in 1976 and 29.8 years in 1977. In the spring of 1977 the Bureau of the Census[1] reported there were 23 million people over 65 years of age (about 10.6% of the 216 million total) and more than 32 million people over 60. By August 1978, the statistics had changed[2] : as of July 1977 there were 32.9 million people over 60, or 15.2% of the resident population, an increase of 15% since 1970. The elderly woman has grown faster than the older man, 17% versus 13%; the percentage of elderly blacks faster than whites, 20% versus 14%. It is expected there may be 29-33 million people over 65 by the 21st Century. One and one quarter million people reach 65 every 50 weeks and 1 of every 8 Americans is 65 or over; in the 21st Century 1 in 5 could be 65 years or older.

LIFE EXPECTANCY

In the year 2050, the Bureau of the Census[1] predicts that life expectancy at birth for women in this country will

---

[1] (released in July 1977—reported in L.A. Times, July 26, 1977) Bureau of Census 'Projections of the Population in the United States: 1977 to 2050: DHEW Publication Series P25,
[2] Statistical Notes. National Clearinghouse on Aging, Aug. 1978, pg. 1

1

be 81 years (now 76.5) and for men, 71.8 years of age (now 68.7). It would appear that not only do older persons make up a sizeable percentage of the population today, but they will continue the dramatic increase since the turn of the century when only 3.1 million (4%) Americans were over 65 out of a total of 76 million people.

MOBILITY, MORBIDITY, MORTALITY

Older persons tend to have more and longer hospital stays, almost twice as many and twice as long as younger persons, averaging about 12 days.[2] Males experience longer stays than females in each of the age groups, except in the under 17 and over 65.[3] Older persons see their doctors 50% more often, (6.6 visits for persons 75 years and over) and live through more days of disability. They spend more on drugs, especially those used for the chronic conditions more prevalent among older people. Fewer acute conditions are reported by people over 45 years of age each year, men reporting fewer problems than women. For a small minority, long term facilities may serve as 'residence' for one time or another during the later years. About 15% of 45-64 year olds are hospitalized each year and about 25% of those over 65. Yet 83% of the 65+ group reported no hospitalization in the year from 1974-1975.

Mortality tables, informative and necessary as they are, are limited in what can be learned about health changes and trends with age. Two recent reports, one from the National Center for Health Statistics (1974), and the first annual report to Congress from HEW, (January, 1976)[4] suggest more accurately the dynamics of health in the nation. Important changes are in the making.

---

[2] from Current Estimates, Health Interview Survey, U.S. 1975 DHEW Publication Number (HRA) 77-1543 (Public Health Service, Health Resources Administration).

[3] from Vital and Health Statistics; data from the National Health Survey, Prevalence of Chronic Conditions. U.S. 1973. Series 10 #109, DHEW Pub. No. (HRA) 77-1536 Pg. 3 March 1977.

[4] Health, United States, 1975, DHEW Pub. No. (HRA) 76-1232.

COMMON CAUSES OF DEATH IN MIDDLE AGE AND OLD AGE

Total deaths between ages:	45-64	65+
Cardiovascular	39%	50%
Cancer	24%	15%
Hypertension	7%	15%
Respiratory	5%	6%
Accidents	5%	2%

All other causes are much less frequent — (adapted from 1968 Vital Statistics of the U.S.)

About 81% of the aged in communities have no limitations on their mobility, 14% have no known chronic disease, but 67% do. However, 17.6% have some trouble getting around, 7% need the help of another person, 6% require help of some type of special equipment or aid and about 5% are homebound. It appears that about 95% of older Americans do live within communities and depend on community resources and services for the maintenance of a life style, and indeed for survival. However, by 85 and older, 19% are residents of institutions.[5]

HEALTH AND DISEASE/HEALTH EXPENDITURES

There does appear to be increased vulnerability to disease with age. Thus, superimposed on the years, are the major chronic diseases — the three major causes of death at any age, cardiovascular disorders, cancer, stroke. Other chronic degenerative diseases also increase with age — atherosclerosis, arthritis, rheumatism, emphysema and hypertension. Nevertheless, there are old people everywhere who are relatively free of disease. A majority of older persons report themselves in good health in spite of the presence of one or more chronic diseases. It is therefore a simplistic assumption that underlies the oft repeated notion that aging is disease or that 'getting old' is inevitably 'getting sick' (Weg 1975, 1976).

---

[5] Health, United States, 1975, DHEW Pub. No. (HRA) 76-1232.

The stereotypes of aging, the relegation to helpless, dependent, asexual and invalid status still dominate our thinking, planning and practices. This is no accident, and has come about as a result of early studies which compared well, college age youth to ill, institutionalized elderly. The 'sick' image of age is a pervasive idea and difficult to unseat, though it has outlived the reality for a majority of older persons.

Although only 10.6% of the population, more than 29% of all health expenditures are made in behalf of persons over 65 today (July, 1977). Costs[6] for health care of the over 65 are not only greater, but have increased at a greater rate. For example, in 1973, $300 per person was spent for those under 65 and increased to $330 FY 1974. In the 19-64 group, FY 75 was up to $492/capita, and rose to $547 in FY 76. For those 65, the 1973 health care costs amounted to $1,052 and to $1,218 for FY 1974 — an increase of over 30%. In FY 1975, 65 and over expenses had risen to $1,335.72 and continued to increase for FY 1976 to $1,521.36 per person. Health, as perceived by older persons, appears to be maintained at better levels than generally assumed. It has been estimated that more than 66% of Americans over 65 say their health is good or excellent, about 22% describe health as fair, and only 9% feel their health is poor.[7] If there is only marginal success in some of the biomedical studies now in progress, if only some headway is made in reducing the incidence of the chronic diseases — then there may be 70% of the 65 and over group who should be able to describe their health as good.

A recently completed survey by the National Institute of Senior Centers reports that 33% of the Senior Centers provide health services in addition to other services.[8] There

---

[6] Gibson, R.M., Mueller, M.S. National Health Expenditures, FY 1976 from Social Security Bulletin, HEW Publication No. (SSA) 77-11700, April, 1977.

[7] Health, United States, 1975, DHEW Pub. No. (HRA) 76-1232.

[8] Memo, National Institute of Senior Citizens (Program of National Council on the Aging, Inc.) May, 1976.

are in excess of 1000 information and referral and counseling programs; 589 centers offer screening services; 411 immunization services; 368 have a nurse part-time; 126 have nurse full time and 135 have a physician part-time. Numbers of Centers are in the process of developing home health services for the frail elderly and for regular participants. It is this kind of programming which may reach the 24% of older persons who have never had a physical examination because typical clinics are threatening.

AGING IS NOT A DISEASE — PHYSIOLOGICAL EFFICIENCY DIMINISHES SLOWLY (Weg, 1975, 1976)

In spite of the attention to chronic diseases and dysfunctions that accompany the years, aging itself — a reflection of the many molecular, cellular and systemic processes that take place with time, is not a disease!

It is useful to acknowledge what physiological differences do occur, and examine their importance. There are many changes in appearance and function that are observable and measurable with age;[9] the wrinkling skin, graying, thinning hair and slower gait. Vision grows less acute (many wear glasses), audition diminishes, stamina and strength decline — the muscle mass is less, and what remains may be visibly flabby, fat tissue increases. The skeletal frame appears and becomes smaller, the person is shorter with age and finger joints have enlarged. Men and women aged 45-79 have a greater prevalence and severity of periodontal problems than the average for all adults 18-79. Average number of decayed, missing, or filled teeth increases with age in both sexes.

Other decrements and modifications are not so easily seen but may be even more significant to basic health maintenance. The capacity for homeostasis — the return of the responsive body to a pre-stress or pre-stimulus level, slowly decreases with age in its efficiency and speed of attainment. At rest, body temperature, blood volume, blood

---

[9] All of the physiological cellular and molecular changes with time are examined in greater detail in references: Weg 1975, 1976.

levels of glucose and amino acids, electrolytes and pH are relatively constant with the advancing years. Many older individuals exhibit blood pressures and heart rates that compare relatively well with younger persons — but again, only at rest. Stress exposes the declining ability to achieve responses equivalent to the earlier years, to a variety of emotional and physical stimuli. Increased time is required to restore pre-stress measurements. It would appear, that the younger individual is characterized by a considerable reserve and redundancy in tissue and organ system capacity (Shock, 1974). With death and dysfunction of cells over time, redundancy is minimized and reserve dwindles. As the reduction in reserve capacity continues and demands of the environment (internal and external) can no longer be adequately met with regularity and predictability, pathology may follow.

Important systemic functions are increasingly marked by a decrease in efficiency. Decreases in maximum breathing capacity, residual lung volume, total capacity and basal oxygen consumption — all contribute to a diminished metabolic rate. The kidney demonstrates some loss of the ability to concentrate urine. Alterations without pathology in the cardiovascular system are measurable: cardiac output and stroke index decrease, whereas peripheral resistance, circulation time, and systolic blood pressure increase in the majority of older persons. Hormonal changes are also measurable, but the data are equivocal. However, clearly decreasing levels of sex hormones are reported for older men and women.

The nervous system also exhibits some changes, some of which are translated into altered behavior. Although simple reflex time remains relatively constant from 20 to 80 years, reaction time shows significant decline with the years, involving a complex of factors in the central nervous system as well as a number of synapses. Any age-related decline in overall function of the nervous system had earlier been assigned to the apparent loss of postmitotic neurons. However, it appears the most rapid loss of neurons occurs between birth and maturity — and the loss after maturity proceeds at a very low level. Diminished neuronal capacity may also be secondary to non-neuronal alterations and dysfunction in blood flow, tissue permeability, connective tissue and responsivity of receptors. Digestive juices are lower in volume, and the rate of peristalsis is down. Meeting the challenges of a variety of diseases is the primary responsibility of the immune system, which also grows less responsive and less efficient. Antibody synthesis decreases quantitatively and qualitatively. The hormones of the thymus and thyroid glands, prime movers in the immune processes, are either lower in concentration or are unable to locate enough appropriate receptors on target tissues, thereby reducing or eliminating the hormonal activities. The response mounted is less effective in resisting e.g. cancer cell development. An increase in 'pathologic' autoimmune bodies may also be a factor in the destruction of body tissues and the development of autoimmune diseases.

On the cellular and molecular levels, many changes with age have been reported. One finds differences in enzyme activities − some increase, some decrease. Serum and tissue ionic balance of calcium, potassium, sodium is not easily maintained. There are suggestions that with age, brain bioamines, the neurotransmitters which carry messages from neuron to neuron, are altered both in concentration and activities. Cellular deterioration is frequently noted in the increasing numbers of aberrant mitochondria and/or fewer mitochondria, disrupted lysosomal and cellular membranes and abnormal nuclei. Connective tissue, the interstitial substance which is largely collagen, crosslinks and become less soluble.

What is most characteristic of aging decrements is the gradual nature of the decline. Homeostatic balances continue to be achieved though at different levels. Without frank pathology, the changes are so gradual as to leave the person largely unaware. Even more particularly related to older persons is their uniqueness − they grow more different from one another with the years. Moreover, no two people age in the same way at the same rate. There is no unified rate of change that is the same for all the tissues and organ systems in the same individual. There is no 'the aged' − this in spite of the necessity for making generalizations in the preparation of materials for publication and/or presentation. Perhaps the most relevant observation for the understanding of the aging population today is that with all the decrements identified, the majority of older persons cope relatively well with the demands of everyday life. With each cohort, they do so more effectively — supported by more education, better health. Most recently, the older person appears to be developing an increasing sense of self as a continuum, so that old becomes, not the 'useless invalid' of the negative stereotype, but another life stage in which challenges, rewards and continued growth are possible.

Normal aging covers the variety of changes with time briefly touched on in the preceding pages. These changes will be expressed in quite different patterns among peoples of this country (and the world) and develop from the interaction of genetic history, resistance to disease, physical activity, diet, a host of social and phychological factors e.g. stress, alienation, loneliness, poverty, etc. Aging is not disease. Remaining vigorous, mobile and active in the later years is realizable. Exercise, good nutrition, adequate interpersonal involvement and minimal negative stress have been implicated in improving the ability to fight disease and the achievement of a sense of well being. Fortunately, this path to good health is, in part, in the hands of the middle aged and older person. On society's part the commitment to older persons becomes more evident — the mythology and stereotypes are slowly crumbling — and those over 65 emerge as whole persons with promise for continuing contribution. What also emerges is the fragmentary nature of our knowledge, related to the concept of 'health and age' rather than 'disease and age'. This points to the necessity for designing aging research in terms of human needs and capacities and using the information to bring about necessary changes.

The disease model of aging is no longer functional for the long pull, in face of the phenomenal increase in older persons, and will certainly be less useful as we move into the 21st century. What may be more in keeping with the potential 17% of a population over 65 in the 21st century are the 'well people clinics' with the kind of objectives that realize: the maintenance of vigor and the prevention of disease, early detection and treatment of even the mildest disorder, attention to total life style. The benefits could be great – the gain to society of the valuable human reserve in energy and talent, of financial resources not needed for custodial care. The gain to individuals is continued growth of capacities and personality, unfettered by debilitating disease.

NUTRITION
its perceived importance in history and today

HISTORY

The belief in the special magic of foods may go back to the days when Eve convinced Adam to bite the apple and know good and evil. Egyptians fed garlic to the workmen on the great pyramids because they were convinced it strengthened the body. On the other hand, according to Herodotus (Greek historian of 5th Century B.C.) the Egyptians believed that all diseases had their origin in food. Therefore, they 'purged' themselves for one day of every month. Discorides, a Greek physician of the first Century A.D. prescribed a potion of grasshoppers to relieve bladder disorders and the liver of an ass to cure epilepsy.

In the search for longevity, some have looked to the steady diet of yogurt of the herdsmen and peasants in Bulgaria and Romania, others to peaches or apricots, symbols of longevity in China. Such nutritional beliefs and fairy tales extend into our contemporary, more scientific age. Food has a long history as one of the tools of medicine. Even in early Greek times, the physician Hippocrates (considered the father of medicine) would prescribe particular diets as part of a therapeutic regimen for his patients, firm in his belief that good health depended upon a particular combination of nutrients (Sebrell and Haggerty, 1967 p. 11).

CURRENT CONCERN

Increasing signs of concern in the society for more adequate nutrition are in the plethora of health food stores, food supplements, countless magazine and newspaper articles about the relationship between food and health, food and longevity, food and sexuality, etc. The very reality of support for food faddism is another expression of the search for an optimum nutrition. An almost subliminal consciousness that "we may be what we eat" appears basic to the hope that food will make us healthy and long lived. Such expectations have encouraged the uninformed 'expert' to capitalize on the widespread ignorance about nutrition among members of the medical profession, researchers and the public at large. In lay magazines as well as scientific journals there is allusion to the concept that a poor diet will shorten life and good nutrition will contribute to the fulfillment of the normal life span. A diet to protect the individual against disease and insure prolonged life has not been designed though correlations abound.

LONG LIVED PEOPLES

Preliminary exploration of the long lived peoples of the world in the highlands of Georgia, of the Soviet Caucasus, the village of Vilcabamba in Ecuador and the principality of Hunza in West Pakistan suggests that the kind and amount of food may be one of the important factors in their advanced age and vigor (Leaf, A. 1973). Even if one accepts the notion that there has been some exaggeration of the age of these peoples, they are advanced in years compared with the average life span of the world's human population. They all share in frugal diets, rich in vegetables and fruits, low in meat and dairy products, low in caloric intake, 1200 to 1900 kcalories compared to our own average 3300 kcalories. Continued record keeping and further investigation of the life span, vitality and activities of these pepoles may provide further clues about the particular parts that nutrition, exercise, attitude toward life, and stress play in the overall life styles represented, in their prolongevity and good health.

AGE AND FOOD: POTENTIAL FOR QUACKERY

Students of child growth and development have long accepted the slowing of growth and development as an early indication of nutritional deficiencies (Tanner, 1973). No experimental evidence exists that age alone produces nutritional problems. Nevertheless, a significant proportion of middle aged and aged today have chronic diseases and/or psychosocial stress which interact with poor nutrition (Smith and Bierman, 1973). Americans are bilked of over one half billion dollars every year by food quackery that appeals to the fears of illness and premature death. Both cynical and sincere promoters of a variety of miracle foods find older people a vulnerable target. However, gerontologists, and the medical profession have generally neglected the possibility that there may be a potentially critical role for adequate nutrition in the quality of life and acceleration of the rate of aging, except in instances of blatant malnutrition and obvious deficiency diseases. The long range, more pervasive effects on larger numbers of middle aged and older people may depend on the probability of extensive subclinical malnutrition.

MALNUTRITION

There are many references to obesity as a problem with increasing age, in face of decreasing physical activity and work role pressure. Although the reserve of energy in adipose tissue has been identified as a possible cause for lower mortality rate of females of all ages during severe food restriction in war ravaged countries, obesity is also considered critically related to hypertension, incidence of cardiovascular disease and cancer. Refined carbohydrates (sucrose) are implicated by many investigators in the morbidity and mortality of older people contributing to increased serum cholesterol, age related lower glucose tolerance, and obesity. However, recent accounts of growing deficiencies among middle aged and older people indicates that both over nutrition and under nutrition require careful investigation.

There are suggestions in the literature that nutrient deficiencies may lead to decreased learning performance, depression, confusion and disorientation. Repeatedly, recent articles and discussions report that low vitamin intake correlates with increased incidence of nervous, circulatory and respiratory disorders. More importantly, perhaps, is that with increased dosage of some vitamins, there was some amelioration of the disorders. Frequently, diagnoses of irreversible brain damage or senility have been made with little regard for the possible nutritional basis for the symptomology. Elderly, disoriented patients assumed to be suffering from cerebral atheroma could be confused because of a vitamin B_{12} deficiency. Vitamin E has been hailed by

some as a panacea in the treatment of a variety of conditions
— circulatory dysfunction, symptoms of menopause, burns,
aberrant fat metabolism and the respiratory effects of
pollutants.

It has also been suggested that vitamin C as an
antioxidant, may play a therapeutic role in the retardation of
aging. But the scientific data are fragmentary and equivocal.
In a study of surviving women, and the death certificates of
those who died, a positive relationship between prior dietary
intake and the age at which death occurs, was found. Those
women with diets rich in ascorbic acid (vitamin C) lived
longer, in agreement with an earlier study among older men
and women of San Mateo County, California. However, the
diet of the survivors was also characterized by a relative
reduction in fat and increased protein consumption. Therefore, it is possible and necessary to consider more than any
one nutrient in the examination of potential 'cause and
effect' data.

Increasingly, minerals receive attention as essential
elements in adequate nutrition. Identified, accepted functions for potassium and sodium in the health and function of
neuronal and muscular tissue are the basis for much
chemotherapy in the treatment of cardiovascular and
neuromuscular difficulties. Other minerals including calcium,
zinc, copper, molybdenum, manganese, selenium and fluoride
are also essential for numerous biochemical reactions in the
body, in greater amounts than heretofore known. The list
will undoubtedly grow longer as our technological vision and
capacity for micromeasurement increases.

The cariogenic nature of sucrose — ingested in large
quantities in childhood and youth — often results in the early
loss of teeth. The loss along with the continued inadequate
nutritional habit patterns in adulthood and middle years
contribute to the widespread periodontal problems which in
turn lead to the edentulous state of many older persons. Real
difficulty with chewing of necessary foods and the consequent diminished pleasure in eating, mark the lives of too
many elderly whose natural dentition is lacking or poor. In
those situations, where prostheses have been substituted,
they are at best an additional source of decreased enjoyment

of eating. Much of this difficulty could be avoided with continued preventive, operative dental care and careful appropriate nutrition earlier in life. Careful eating in the middle and later years remains important for the maintenance of natural dentition which potentiates adequate nutriture in the later years. Otherwise, a circular situation may develop in which poor nutrition may lead to loss of teeth which in turn exacerbates nutritional inadequacy.

Beyond the requirements and function of particular nutrients and the frequently conflicting opinions of the so-called experts concerning dietary regimes — a consideration of nutrition for older persons in health and disease highlights the importance for an individual approach to the nature of food intake. With older people, well or ill, individual differences are even greater. At a time of life when many changes are taking place — diminishing roles as worker and active parent, death of friends and spouses, curtailment of mobility, decreased income, decline in homeostatic efficiency, slowness of response, and increased probability of illness, food gains in significance. For some, food may even be a source of feelings of security. For others, food may become a substitute for the warm human interactions, especially if alienation from the mainstream of living becomes acute. Many elderly who live alone, miss the socializing aspects of eating, do not prepare nutritious meals, and succomb to the malnutrition of the underfed. The low poverty level of the fixed incomes of more than one quarter of older persons in this country exacerbates the malnutrition attributable to loneliness, poor dentition, or ignorance of cookery. Food is expensive today.

The consideration of nutrition and human aging in many of the studies and increasing attention to the multiple interactions among physiology, age, life style, health, disease and nutrition, suggest that nutrition is a major environmental factor in the achievement of longevity, in resistance to infection/disease and in the tolerance and response to stress.

This examination of nutrition and aging will deal primarily with the relationship of nutrition to the structural and functional body changes with time. Although numerous environmental factors are indeed intimately involved in nutritional adequacy and habits, our concern shall be with the dynamic interactions among nutrients, physiological changes with time, pathological alterations, and affective factors.

Jean Mayer's (Mayer, 1974) concept of the relationship of nutrition and aging at three levels succinctly indicates the many variables that interact.

1. Through the greater possibility for disabilities, loneliness, transportation barriers, and decreased income, good nutrition is endangered.

2. Through the participation of malnutrition in the development of disease that accompanies old age.

3. Through the potential, yet undefined effect nutrition may have in affecting the nature and rate of aging.

At yet a fourth level — neglect, ignorance and ratio of patients to attendants in nursing homes address the wide ranging factors that relate to nutritional adequacy. Any complete consideration of nutrition of older persons, or more appropriately, the last half of life, would include variables involved at all four levels.

Roger Williams' (1967) article in NUTRITION TODAY "We Abnormal Normals," reports that in one of his earlier studies he was impressed with the importance of "nutrition individuality": 12 healthy young people were studied using repeated tests related to taste sensitivities, composition of saliva and composition of urine. Not one of the 12 was similar to any average person that may be inferred from RDA values and each one differed from the others. Strong resemblances were identified in only two, and these belonged to a pair of identical twins who were purposely included. Although this study was carried out with a statistically small "N," and a young sample, the data are suggestive. Indeed, one of the primary characteristics of older persons as a population is the growing uniqueness of the individual: in personality and behavior, in physiological changes and in the rate of aging.

It is clear that assessing nutritional status (at any age) is in its infancy, that additional data are necessary from household surveys and the biochemical and clinical consequences of individual nutrient intake. For now, the best estimates of acceptable daily intake are the Recommended Dietary Allowances (RDA), revised and published periodically by the Food and Nutrition Board of the National Research Council. The Board defines the RDA as "levels of intake of essential nutrients considered, on the basis of available scientific knowledge, to be adequate to meet the known nutritional needs of practically all healthy people."[10] Generally, values below RDA level are indicated as 2/3 RDA — low level and 1/3 RDA — deficient level. These levels appear to some clinicians and scientists to be suggestive of nutritional risks (Henderson, 1972).

The RDA values cannot be considered adequate to meet any additional needs of individuals whose energies and metabolites are drained by disease or stress. It is instructive to note that the recommended allowances are calculated for the hypothetical, healthy, reference man, woman, or child. For example: the 'Reference Man' weighs 65-70kg, is 25 years old, free of disease, physically fit for active work, and lives in a temperate climate. He is in caloric balance, works 8 hours a day, is sedentary for 4 hours, may walk for up to 1-1.5 hours in recreation, and is assumed to require on the average 3200 kcalories per day throughout the year.[10,11] Any resemblance of a majority of older persons to the aforementioned characteristics is generally improbable. But, in keeping with the National Research Council definition, the RDA is only an estimated acceptable daily nutrient intake, which can (and should) be modified, adapted to. meet the needs of people with different life-styles, economic levels, cultural food patterns and disease. Nevertheless, the adaptation or modification is rarely undertaken.

---

[10] Recommended Dietary Allowances 8th ed. National Academy of Sciences 1974.

[11] Beaton, G.H., Bengoa, J.M. *Nutrition in Preventive Medicine.* Geneva, World Health Organization, 1976 458-460. See Appendix #.

Most of the evaluations of nutritional adequacy of older persons, in this country and abroad, have been made on the basis of comparison with these hypothetical average values. The very few longitudinal studies cited still use the RDA as the measuring stick. As with the study of physiological changes in the last half of life, what is sorely needed are nutritional values more in keeping with the physiological, pathological, emotional and environmental realities of aging persons. Moreover, in view of the range of individual differences, it is necessary to complete careful physical examinations and biochemical analyses in order to make realistic dietary recommendations.

$\mathcal{C}hanging$
$\mathcal{R}equirements$ 2

Some researchers and clinicians in the field conclude that nutrient requirements change with age, and others with comparable data, state that nutrient requirements do not change with time.

ENERGY EXPENDITURE/ENERGY REQUIREMENTS

Inoye, et al., (1962) of the University of Kyoto, compared young, middle-aged, and old subjects in regard to energy expenditure. They found basal metabolism declined by 8% in the aged. This decline may be more apparent than real if the slow metabolic decrement is viewed in terms of the lean body mass (tissues involved). Due to the accompanying changes in composition of the body — "this decline is not really a decline at all" (Bierman, 1976 p. 171). The percentage of bodily adipose tissue continues to increase with time, with the concomitant decline of muscle tissue and bone. Although exercise and sports may increase muscle mass, there is a decrease in lean body mass at an increasing rate past middle age (Moore et al., 1963; Moore et al., 1968; Novak, 1972). A gradual decrease in total body potassium (K) is a further reflection of the decrease in muscle and bone since K is essentially absent from neutral fat.

Energy expenditure for lying, sitting, standing and walking showed little change with age. However, as suspected, work efficiency declined with age from 37% in the young to 28% in the older group. *It would appear that the older person uses more energy to perform the same amount of work.* (author's emphasis)

ADEQUACY OF DIETARY CALORIES

There frequently exists a direct proportionality between total daily caloric intake, and the ingested amounts of fat, protein, and regulatory nutrients (calcium, iron, thiamin, and vitamin A, etc.). A study of Swedish older men and women with an intake of 1400-2000 kcalories demonstrated this direct relationship: as the kcalories decreased so did protein and the regulatory nutrients. The researcher involved sees this group as nutritionally at risk and facing frank deficiencies unless changes are made (NUTRITION REVIEWS, 1966)[1]

Preliminary findings of diet and biochemical tests in the First Health and Nutrition Examination Survey[2] are that 21% of the white and 36% of the black adults aged 60 and over in the lower income group had daily intakes of less than 1000 kcalories.

Thirty-two healthy American midwestern women living at home (age 65-85) had their diets assessed primarily via dietary history: protein and caloric intake were significantly correlated (Fry et al., 1963). Nearly all of the women ingested at least 2/3 of the RDA (low level) for each nutrient evaluated: protein, calcium, iron, vitamins A, thiamin (B_1), riboflavin (B_2), niacin (B_3) and ascorbic acid (C).

Dr. George Briggs (1974), a professor of nutrition at Berkeley, points to the consequences of the dilution of the diet. With the refining and processing of more and more foods, the character of nutrient intake has changed: usually

---

[1] NUTRITION REVIEWS, 24; 319-20, 1966.

[2] DHEW Public. No. 74-1291-1, 1974, 7-18.

[3] The Roe (1976) book represents a detailed examination of concepts and review of the literature.

with more sodium than needed, and less potassium, zinc, selenium, chromium, silicon, and nickel. Too many extra calories (usually through the addition of sugars and fats) dilute the diet, particularly in relation to minerals and vitamins. Yet, with the reduction of kcalories and total food intake, it becomes increasingly difficult to ingest the necessary amount of regulatory nutrients and dietary fiber.

PROTEINS

The rate of total body protein synthesis was measured comparing infants, young adults, and elderly women, all on adequate diets. Results demonstrated: (1) rate of syntheses declines with age, declining approximately 80% by adult-hood; (2) efficiency of nitrogen utilization showed no marked variation with age. Based on this study, the daily dietary protein requirements declines roughly 30% between age 20 and 75 (Young et al., 1975). Intakes very low in protein are frequently low in vitamins and minerals found in abundance in protein food sources (Mayer, 1974).

Irwin and Hegsted (1971) review the research on protein requirements of older persons and find the literature equivocal. They also find that the age grouping of "65 and over" is inadequate as a basis for comparison. Nutritional needs of an ill, failing 65-year-old could differ significantly from those of an active, energetic 80-year-old. Some early studies appear to indicate a need for a relatively high intake of protein in order to maintain nitrogen equilibrium. They allude to four other studies which come to different conclusions, e.g.: older persons need more protein, need less protein, and the protein requirements of the elderly are not very different from those of younger adults. Irwin and Hegsted's position is essentially in agreement with Miller and Stare (1968) who found the evidence for change of protein requirements with age inconclusive.

There may be hazards involved with the low caloric intake generally recommended for older persons. Based on the assumption that "the aged" are much less active, the decision has been for a decreased caloric diet. This ignores the fact that the muscles and neurons of older persons may function less efficiently, and therefore use more energy to do less work (See earlier ref., Inoue et al., 1962). Due to the low carbohydrate and fat levels that usually accompany the low kcalorie intake, the protein present will be used first for energy production, leaving little protein available to fulfill its customary metabolic role (Durnin, 1968). Durnin suggests that part of the "wasting" of muscle tissue which apparently occurs with aging might be retarded with adequate protein intake.

Dietary nitrogen (N) and the essential amino acids are necessary for the maintenance of organ protein synthesis. Consequently, the total daily requirement will depend on the size and metabolic status of the protein mass (Young et al., 1976). Body N (protein mass) decreases during later years, more rapidly in men than in women (Forbes and Reina, 1970). It would appear then, that total protein requirement of older persons is "less per unit of body weight, but similar per unit of body cell mass when compared with young adults" (Young et al., 1976). Aging does appear to be characterized by a decrease in the amount of total body protein synthesized daily, with relatively greater total body protein syntheses taking place in the viscera (Young et al., 1976).

Young et al., (1976) speculates that since the periphery will need less exogenous amino acids, this might reduce the overall requirement for exogenous sources of N and essential amino acids. Their preliminary findings, based on plasma amino acid levels of tryptophan and valine, suggest that amino acid requirements per unit of body cell mass may be higher in the healthy elderly as compared to young adults.

Most of the studies to estimate protein needs apply to healthy persons. It is reasonable to suggest that reduced efficiency of dietary N could result from altered gastrointestinal activity, infection, and/or the changed metabolic patterns of disease accompanying age in many older persons. The net effect would be a hightened protein requirement.

REGULATORY NUTRIENTS, LOW CALORIE INTAKE AND RDA'S

Iron intake was thought to be marginal in old age, yet Miller and Stare (1968) suggested that iron requirements may indeed increase with age. They noted, too, that appropriate levels (different from the current RDA levels) of vitamin D, calcium, and fluoride need careful attention related to what they call "senile osteoporosis." Schlettwein-Gsell (1966) found no significant difference in micronutrient requirements between the young and the old, and assigned importance to the excessive intake of saturated fats and calories.

Mann (1973) noted, as have many others (Bender, 1971; Exton-Smith, 1972; Whanger, 1973; Mayer, 1974), that older persons require food intake with higher concentration of micronutrients per calorie than younger individuals. This is especially true as the caloric intake decreases. Food intake of 100 white women (40 years of age and over) were measured over a period of time. When 2000 kcalories were eaten each day, nutrients ingested were within the RDA. But when intake was cut to 1000 kcalories, all nutrients ingested were less than 2/3 of the RDA, with the exception of vitamins A and C which relate primarily to the use of fruits and vegetables (Ohlson, 1964).

There are difficulties in the use of the RDA's, both in the interpretation of food consumption data and the planning of diets (Leverton, 1975). Since the margin of safety which has not been included in the RDA is different for different nutrients, a quantitative value for an overall margin of safety has not been provided. Therefore, it is not a simple task to determine at what intake level, lower than the RDA, a person is considered at risk. Many consider the RDA ideal, and assume the values imply average requirements — both assumptions leading to misunderstanding.

Dr. Hegsted (1975a) of the Harvard School of Public Health is also critical of the use of the RDA. He is of the opinion that the recommended dietary allowance cannot be equally useful to plan diets, and to purchase food supplies, as well as to determine the adequacy of nutrition from food consumption data. He later (Hegsted, 1975b) notes that most experimental studies on nutritional requirements yield only an estimation of the *mean requirement* (author's emphasis) of the group or groups under study. It is clear that such values could not relate specifically to as much as half of the population. A telling and generally ignored point he makes relates to his observation of the mounting evidence of

interaction between and among nutrients as well as interaction of food with drugs. Critical of the method of
obtaining food intake information, he notes that the 24-hour
food recall is too limited to be representative of eating habits,
and recall without third party observation, may be too
inaccurate. Changing requirements may be even greater than
are warranted by the changing physiology of aging, primarily
as a function of the processing, packaging, and mass
preparation of foods.

Dr. Schroeder confirms (Lear, 1970) the claims made by
Turner (1970) in *THE CHEMICAL FEAST* that of the
approximately two dozen nutrients removed from bread and
other cereal products only four are restored vitamins, thiamin
(B_1), riboflavin (B_2), niacin (B_3) and iron. Added iron's
usefulness is questionable since it is in the ferric form not
easily absorbed by the body. In addition, the FDA standards
for baked goods permits 93 different ingredients, few of
them nutrients, to be added to bread products at the
discretion of the processors. None of the ninety-three
additives is required to be listed on the label. It must be
remembered that these foods are not expected to be the sole
items of the diet, and therefore are not required to provide
all of the daily required nutrients.

Although a number of the references indicate that older
persons require higher concentrations of vitamins and
minerals per kcalorie intake, there are few studies which have
been done to provide precise data. It would be particularly
meaningful if long term regimens of some of the nutrients in
question were instituted. This has been done in short term
studies, e.g., iron, reported elsewhere in this monograph.
Accumulated, continuing measurements and records of food
intake, blood levels, functions of particular systems and
overall health would be invaluable. Both subjective and
observer records would be necessary.

FOOD/DRUG INTERACTIONS

There is no doubt that drugs are 'double edged swords'
in relation to human health and disease. Necessary and often
life saving, drugs may be unexpectedly hazardous, also
potential causes of disease, illness, invalidism and even death

(Cohen, 1975; Davidson, 1973; Exton-Smith and Windsor, 1971). In the last few years, there is evidence of a growing awareness of the special factors that must be considered in the prescription and use of drugs for the older person (Roe, 1976; Weg, 1973).

It is reasonable that, in view of the changing physiology with time and the numbers of drugs typically prescribed (and/or taken) for the middle and older patient, there needs to be a different regimen for drug use than in the earlier years. Chronic and progressive diseases are more common and any apparent crisis may be due to an acute phase of a chronic disease or to a piling up of effects of the multiple diseases that co-exist. Pharmacological intervention often proves to be an exacerbation of existing symptoms and/or the development of a new disorder, heretofore not present — iatrogenesis (Davison, 1973). Possible alterations in gastrointestinal absorption, changes in proportions of lean body mass and fat, receptor sites for drug molecules, circulatory and metabolic modification, changes in liver, excretory and homeostatic functional capacities may be significantly involved in drug response, all or in part, in a single individual (Weg, 1973). Moreover, drug interaction and idiosyncratic drug response may present additional problems since both appear to increase with age and intensify the hazards of drug therapy in older persons (Davison, 1973; Modell, 1974). Major attention in this examination is with the interaction between nutrients and drugs that may interfere with effective, necessary reactions of each, and most particularly with drug-induced nutritional deficiencies. The effects on nutrition range from the dramatic (nausea, vomiting) to the more subtle: altered sense of taste, anorexia, use and metabolic rate of absorbed nutrients, their transport, storage and elimination (Hartshorn, 1977; Pawan, 1974; Roe, 1976).[3]

If inadequate nutrition in one or more nutrients is present in the older person (with lack of obvious apparent symptoms), any additional stress on the nutritional status

---

[1] National Center for Health Statistics, Public Health Service, (1966).

created by drug/nutrient interactions may result in the clinical symptomology of malnutrition. Drugs may displace nutrients from plasma protein or tissue binding sites by either combining with the nutrient, competitively replacing nutrients on the receptor site, or a combination of both (Roe, 1976). In the course of drug metabolism, Roe suggests that "structurally unrelated drugs can also stimulate cellular catabolism and reduce body stores of fat soluble and water soluble vitamins." It is also true that maintenance of adequate nutrition could not only increase in individual's tolerance to a drug, but make possible higher dosages when necessary (March, 1976). Drugs can, therefore, increase nutrient requirements at various levels, unless the requirements are fulfilled with an altered dietary intake. One of the most common nutritional effects is in the development of, or exacerbation of hypovitaminoses. Generally, drug-related hypovitaminoses comes about gradually over long periods (Roe, 1976), more probable in the elderly who are chronic rather than occasional users of drugs. Some of the drug's effects on nutritional adequacy which are relevant to older persons include:

hypovitaminosis:
1. Tissue depletion of ascorbic acid can take place under the influence of a number of drugs: alcohol, anorectic agents, atracyclene and aspirin (Coffee & Wilson 1975). Aspirin may be the most important since it is used so widely among all ages, but more often among older persons as a pain reductant. Aspirin also blocks the uptake of ascorbic acid into blood platelets *in vitro* (Sahud, 1970).

2. There are a range of drug therapies fairly common among older adults, that affect the B complex vitamins, in requirements, absorption, utilization and excretion.
   • Requirements for thiamin may be increased in persons using a digitalis alkaloid frequently prescribed in coronary insufficiency or decompensation (Roe, 1976).
   • Drugs that can cause vitamin B_6 deficiency are, hydralazine used in the treatment of hypertension and L-dopa in the treatment of Parkinson's disease.

Phenobarbital, the diuretic triamterene and aspirin affect folate utilization. Since vitamin B_6 is essential at several steps in the syntheses of the vitamin niacin, of neurotransmitters and neurohormones (serotinin, gamma-aminobutyric acid and epinephrine), deficiency results not only in niacin deficiency, but also in neurological symptoms (Roe, 1976).

- Vitamin B_{12} absorption is decreased or inhibited with the use of the biguanides, oral hypoglycemic drugs in the treatment of diabetes (Tomkin, 1973).

3. Absorptive capacity changes of the gastrointestinal tract is measurable as a result of the laxative, mineral oil and an antibiotic.

- Mineral oil, a long-time laxative favorite of many older persons has adverse effects on the absorption of carotene, vitamins A, D and K (Roe, 1976). It has been suggested that the mineral oil may interfere with micelle formation of A, D and K. An alternative explanation (as with carotene) depends upon the solubility of these vitamins in the mineral oil which stimulates excretion of the dissolved vitamins rather than their absorption. Cummings (1974) notes that abuse of cathartics, still in very widespread use (and therefore a public health problem) has caused severe malabsorption syndromes.
- Within 6 hours after the first does of the antibiotic neomycin, absorptive capacity is altered (Keusch et al., 1970). Neomycin therapy results in the decrease of pancreatic lipase (Mehta et al., 1964).

mineral deficiencies:

1. Antacids containing aluminum inhibit intestinal absorption of flouride and phosphorous, increase the excretion of calium in urine and stool with concurrent hypophosphatemia. If this treatment is prolonged, significant skeletal demineralization may occur (Lotz et al., 1968). Among older persons such demineralization may aggravate any tendency to osteomalacia or osteoporosis. (See later discussion of calcium metabolism and osteoporosis).

2. Long term diuretic therapy for cardiac failure may lead to magnesium deficiency. Patients studied by Lim and Jacob (1972) had been on combined therapy with digoxin, chlorthiazide and furosemide. In their judgement, the magnesium deficiency resulted from "inadequate diets associated with anorexia, as well as administration of the diuretics" (Roe, 1976).

3. An interesting, apparently suggestive effect of diuretics on zinc tissue and serum levels was pursued by Wester (1975). He found that serum zinc levels were lower in 96 non treated healthy subjects than in 210 patients treated for more than 6 months. Wester theorized this could be a function of the decreased blood volume produced by the diuretics. However, the zinc content of liver tissue in autopsies, was lower in the diuretic treated group than in controls. Although it is possible that these tissue differences may be due to different causes of death, Wester views the zinc depletion as most probably related to the diuretic therapy.

Although there is some documentation of drug-induced malnutrition, the numbers of subjects under study have been notably small. Studies of population of older persons, both in the communities and institutions could provide data about nutritional status and the long term use of drugs.

Roe (1976) points to the need for more careful investigation and dissemination of information on incidence, etiology and risk of such malnutrition to allied health professions. Many in the medical and allied health professions were students in the country's medical schools and colleges at a time when most drugs in current use were not on the 'drawing board,' and the dynamics of drug use and abuse was in its infancy. In the education of these professionals, aging and the aged were minimally discussed, nutrition as a significant partner in human health was also neglected (Butler, 1975; Mayer, 1975 b, p. 366).

Physicians frequently depend on the descriptive literature in the complimentary packages of drug items, or on the advice of pharmaceutical 'detail men.' As a group, they remain largely unaware of the compounding effects of the polypharmacy in the treatment of older persons. The multiple drugs are often not only inefficacious for the alleviation of the presenting symptoms, but inimical to adequate nutrition and finally to mental and physical health maintenance.

Recent exposure by governmental agencies of drug abuse among elderly in nursing homes, is only the tip of the iceberg (U.S. Senate Hearings, 1975). The largest numbers of middle aged and older persons are in the communities, their nutrition and health assaulted daily with overmedication or otherwise faulty drug regimens. It is true that older persons (in the community) who are drug abusers do not come to public attention to the degree that younger persons do. More importantly, most common misuse of drugs among older persons appears to be related to those drugs prescribed for them (Peterson and Whittington, 1977).

Most currently, governmental agencies in their recognition of the inadequate, negative position of aging in medical education, would appear to have touched the conscience of the medical profession with promise of funding (Butler, 1975). A few excellent residency programs in geriatrics have been established in the United States (Michelmore, 1975). Schools of Pharmacy are re-examining their curricula (Cheung, 1977). Recent conferences of the Gerontological Society, and meetings of the Medical Colleges of America have specifically addressed the issue of introduction of the concepts of aging, not only as brief topics in other courses, but with possible Chairs of Geriatrics in mind. Among these concepts are nutrition and drugs, their interaction, interdependence; how these change with time. Movement has begun . . . at this writing the Medical School at Cornell University has such a Chair, and the Medical School at the University of Pennsylvania has the question under serious consideration. The importance of such educational change is not only in the sensitization of the medical profession, but in the changed attitudes and practices which will affect the degree and kind of health maintenance of older persons.

STRESS/NUTRITIONAL STATUS/ILLNESS

In a number of studies and reviews, there are indications that life changes (stress) may be significant in their effects on the physiology and health of all persons. Particuarly appropriate to older persons are the suggestions that the demands on the body during stressful periods may not only lead to nutritional imbalance, but lead to illness and finally may affect the rate of age changes (Moss, 1973; Rahe et al., 1970; Seyle, 1970).

There was established a highly significant correlation between life change scores and chronic disease (leukemia, cancer, heart attack, schizophrenia, menstrual difficulties and warts). On a "Social Readjustment Rating Scale," a 75% correlation was demonstrated between the severity of the illness and the number of life change units (Holmes and Masuda, 1972; Rahe et al., 1970). Similar correlations have been validated among pregnant women, leukemia patient families and retirees.

The reality of the multiple changes that older persons experience in American contemporary society (psychologically, socially and physiologically) suggests that mounting stress could tax coping and homeostatic capacities. A breakdown of adaptability (with nutrient imbalance as only one factor) increases the vulnerability to illness, disease and death.

Examples of biochemical changes in blood chemistry have been measured in a number of different situations. Dr. Stewart Wolf of University of Texas, as part of an experiment, moved conversations to stressful topics and found serum cholesterol had increased (Tanner, 1976). Nicotine in cigarette smoke acts as a stimulant to the nervous system which releases the stress hormone, norepinephrine, which in turn elevates blood pressure and releases cholesterol to the blood stream.

Dr. Lennart Levi (1975) showed that quite small changes in the emotional climate or in interpersonal relationships can produce marked changes in body chemistry: urine analysis finds adrenalin increases about 70%, and noradrenaline increases about 35%, catecholamine measurements also varied (rose and fell) with different film clips.

Such repeated insults to the physiology speed up fat metabolism, and decreases glucose tolerance, both already measurably different (from earlier years) in older persons.

Another interesting factor in the stress/nutrition equation is exercise. Viewed by many exercise physiologists and researchers as a basic stress relief measure, regular exercise apparently decreases the stress level, evidenced by a decrease in cholesterol concentrations, blood pressure and blood clotting rate (Carruthers 1974). Extra fats and sugars released into the bloodstream under emotional and/or physical stress can be dissipated by physical exercise. Rate of metabolism, and disposition of metabolite products of nutrient digestion are then, not only a function of available enzymes, energy for catabolism and synthesis, but also of another environmental factor — exercise, under individual control.

Emotional stress is believed to have negative nutritional effects, particularly on nitrogen (N) and calcium (Ca) balance (Elek, 1970; Levi, 1971). Measurements during stress applicable to the evaluation of nutritional status need to become part of as many studies of older persons as possible. Much more data are required before a cause and effect relationship can be firmly established between stress and nutritional deficiencies.

Nutritional Adequacy 3

INCIDENCE OF OVERWEIGHT AND OBESITY

Some geriatricians believe that overweight among older persons rather than undernutrition is the greater problem (Bender, 1971). Even in women over 80, it has been noted that 20% were overweight (Corless, 1973). Though overnutrition is not a major issue in clinical geriatrics, the frequently associated atheromatous degeneration and osteoarthritis are.

In England, the survey by the Department of Health (Corless, 1973) revealed that 53 of 1,367 geriatric patients were obese. Dibble et al., (1967) in an American survey reported that 45 out of 67 elderly females and 12 out of 26 older males were more than 10% overweight. Another American survey (Morgan, 1959), showed "that 40-50% of elderly women and 32% of the men were overweight, while much smaller percentage were underweight; 9% of the women and 19% of the men were 10% more underweight. Neil Solomon (1969) judged that "1 in 5 Americans is overweight, i.e., more than 10% over ideal weight." An obese population has an unusual concentration of afflictions. Two hundred and sixty (260) of the original overweight 541 subjects (nearly half) had one or more of the conditions listed below:

> diabetes mellitus (183); arthritis (127); heart disease (87); gout (75); hypertension (61); kidney disease (52); hypercholesteremia (44); hernia (41); thyroid disease (29); colitis (15); peptic ulcer (7); cancer (3); other conditions (27).

It would appear that the percentage of persons that are 20% or more above 'best' weight increases with age up to a point, and then drops, close to the 6th decade (Goodhart and Shils, 1973). Females arrive at a maximum average weight between ages 55-64, and males between 35-54.[1]

	Males	Females
20 - 29 years	12%	12%
50 - 59 years	34%	46%
60 - 69 years	29%	45%

Obesity is considered an ongoing metabolic and physiological reflection of a number of processes and results in the accumulation of fat cells. There appears to be widespread agreement that obesity develops, related in the beginning to genetic individuality, continued later with a caloric intake greater than caloric expenditure (Fox, 1973; Heald, 1972; Mayer, 1968; McCracken, 1966; Nelson, 1973). Genetic potential may be fulfilled, modified or enhanced by environment. The work of Hirsch and Knittle (1970) supports the thesis that patterns of nutrition initiated in early childhood, possibly *in utero*, may "stimulate the formation of adipocytes," which proscribes the framework for future obesity. This metabolic status at an early age frequently is maintained and is difficult to alter.

However, it is not at all clear how important size and number of adipose cells are in cause, development, and treatment of obesity, or whether early onset of obesity is more serious than that which starts in adult life (Widdowson and Dauncey, 1976). There appear to be methodological

---

[1] National Center for Health Statistics, Public Health Service, (1966).

concerns that limit the conclusions that can be drawn:

1. A potential adipose cell or preadipocyte and mature adipose cells which have been depleted of lipid cannot be distinguished from other connective tissue cells and therefore are not counted.

2. With current methods, an adipose cell can be identified only when it contains a minimum amount of lipid.

Further, no evidence really exists to establish "a correlation between total number of adipose cells and the degree of obesity or that cellularity of adipose tissue influences the rate of weight reduction produced by a low energy intake" (Widdowson and Dauncey, 1976).

Contrary to earlier beliefs, the number of adipose cells in the adult (in adult onset obesity) may increase and is not fixed (Salans et al., 1973). It has also been demonstrated that preadipocytes of obese adults have greater potential for multiplication in vitro than do those from lean persons (Ng et al., 1971).

The fact that success in many cases of dietary and chemical treatment of obesity is not very permanent is amply documented in the medical literature. A short-lived loss of a few pounds is frequently regained after a year or two or more (Mayer, J., 1965; McCuish, et al., 1968; Stunkard and McLaren-Hume, 1959).

English researchers have focused on the contribution of refined carbohydrate (sucrose) in the morbidity and mortality among older persons (Bender and Damji, 1971; Yudkin and Szanto, 1970; Yudkin, 1972). They have found that sucrose:

1. Increases the level of serum cholesterol, thereby adding to the vulnerability to cardiovascular attack.

2. Exhausts the pancreas leading to maturity-onset diabetes in a percentage of older persons.

3. Contributes to the metabolic patterns for obesity.

Although severe obesity as measured by skinfold thickness appears to be relatively rare in the older age group, the degree of adiposity increases with age (Brozek, 1956). Generally, obesity develops gradually and, if a careful history is taken, its onset can be correlated with a particular landmark such as puberty. Obesity may also develop over a shorter period − 2 to 3 years, following the interruption of "normal" weight control as in pregnancy, childbirth, or surgery. Affective concerns or acute psychological stress may also antedate a period of marked weight gain (McCracken, 1966).

In studies pursued at the Mayo Clinic (Nelson et al., 1973) it became clear (1) that there was a lowered caloric requirement with age, (2) that when exercise is constant, obesity may develop with age even if nutrient intake is somewhat less. West et al., (1970) have suggested that no matter the source of the calories, adiposity is the primary environmental factor responsible for the prevalence of maturity-onset diabetes.

WEIGHT CONTROL: DIET THERAPY; DRUGS; BEHAVIOR MODIFICATION

Dr. Ralph Nelson, (1974) head of clinical nutrition at Mayo Clinic, blames overnutrition for reducing the life span. Animal studies have shown that protein and kcalorie restrictions extend life (McCay, 1935; Ross, 1964). Further there is some evidence that such restrictions in animals result in the decreased and delayed incidence of the degenerative diseases associated with the last half of life (Fanestil and Barrows, 1965; McCay, 1955; Sinclair, 1953).

Animal studies have demonstrated that "conditions for modifying lifespan beneficially appears to be highly critical and age dependent" (Ross, 1972). Feeding programs and diets (with rats), conducive to long life, are most efficient when begun at weaning time, and decreasingly so with age. Those rats that were underfed 7 weeks after weaning and permitted *ad libitum* feeding at 70 days of age, had lower mortality rates than those rats with the same diet content *ad libitum* from 21 days forward. There is in these rats an inverse relationship between lifespan and quantity of food intake which holds only for the first half of life (Ross and Bras, 1971, 1974).

Nelson (1974) has said "no one has shown that weight loss is greater on a protein or carbohydrate restricted diet yet." Weight loss, he believes, is a function of total caloric reduction — not the decline of a single nutrient such as carbohydrate, fat or protein. Efforts at weight reduction among the middle-aged and older persons have frequently been combined with an attack on high cholesterol levels. Yet Nelson's conviction is that "polyunsaturated fats do not reduce blood cholesterol in individuals who have this problem." Other dietary intervention studies (Hazzard and Knopp, 1976) have demonstrated that in free living subjects observed for 10 months diets rich in polyunsaturated fats and low in cholesterol reduced cholesterol a little more than 10%. Confined subjects were followed for 5 years, and demonstrated a 15-16.5% lowering of serum cholesterol.

There is some suggestion in the literature that high levels of polyunsaturates may be harmful, probably carcinogenic (Pearce and Dayton, 1971). It has been demonstrated that there is a correlation between an increase of free radicals and disrupted cell membranes, and increased cross linking of the large, critical protoplasmic molecules — protesins and nucleic acids. Though cause and effect cannot be thus established, the evidence suggests the increased free radicals from the polyunsaturates may result in the described damage.

Weight control and the sought-for weight reduction attempted by drugs alone are short-lived, and possibly dangerous, depending on the individual's general state of health and length of use. However, a number of researchers consider it moderately appropriate to make careful, limited use of anorexigenic drugs. These drugs may be helpful as a part of a program that works towards the development of motivation, educates the individual about diet, good nutrition, and the consequences (short term and long range) of weight gain and weight loss (Fineberg, 1962; Fineberg, 1972; Modell, 1960).

The most recent approach to the treatment of obesity has emphasizes on behavior modification. A number of studies have reported significant weight loss with procedures from experimental psychology (Mahoney, 1974; Stuart, 1967; Stunkard, 1972). Primary effort is expended on "teaching the obese person how to modify one's eating pattern" (Leon, 1974; Stuart and Davis, 1971). The learning approach to weight control is based on boredom, emotional arousal, and anxiety-producing situations (Leon and Chamberlain, 1973 a,b). The goal of behavior modification in this instance: that the overweight and/or obese person learns to limit eating to times and places in keeping with physiological needs.

Weight control — the avoidance of over-or underweight is a legitimate concern with older persons, since both augur a variety of problems for the individual.

Malnutrition may be present in either situation. It would appear quite plain that, on the average, weight control requires accurate knowledge about nutrition and diet, about consequences of drug supplementation and the extreme faddist panaceas. Above all, it may require the conviction that eating less but better is not only possible, but necessary in appropriate weight control.

MEAL SPACING/NUTRITION

For the past 10 to 15 years, there has been increased attention to the spacing and rate of nutrient intake. There are suggestions from some of the experimentation that these variables may result in significant differences in intermediary metabolism and eventual body composition.

It was shown that individuals whose eating pattern was modified "from 3-meals-a-day hospital diet to a formula diet administered six times daily" experienced a decrease in serum cholesterol independent of the nature of the dietary fat (Burton, 1965). Cohn (1961, 1964) noted that the level of serum lipids was lowered if the same diet was divided into a number of small portions.

Irwin and Feeley (1967) observed that the mean serum cholesterol level was lower in 15 healthy women "when diet was served in 3-meals/day than when diet was served in one large or two small meals." In another study 440 men (60-64 years old), representative of that age group in the Prague district (Czechoslovakia), were divided into sub-groups according to the number of daily meals they ate. Results clearly indicated that with the increase in meal frequency, overweight, hypercholesterolemia and diminished glucose tolerance tend to decrease (Fabry et al., 1964). A more recent study by Fabry et al., (1968) showed that in an additional 1,359 men (60-64 years) belonging to the same population group as the earlier investigation, the percentage of subjects with diagnosed ischemic heart disease decreased markedly with increased meal frequency. The decrease was substantial, from 30.4% in the group with an infrequent meal pattern to 19.9% in that sub-group eating five or more meals each day.

LOW-CALORIE FOODS; POTENTIAL FOR NON-STANDARD FOODS

The production and use of low-calorie foods by people across the country and in industrialized European countries have increased (Kreiger, 1973). It appears that acceptability and purchase of such foods depends on "palatability, convenience, and price" much more than on their nutritional value. However, for the clinician, the researcher and older persons, the salient question remains: "How nutritious is it?"

Dietetic foods are defined as "foods used for special conditions such as . . . overweight or old age." Supplemented foods such as tiger's milk are among those included in the definition. Many such dietetic foods are more expensive. As low-calorie foods (a class of dietetic foods) become more customary, it may be important to regulate this industry to assure adequate nutrients in the products. Low-calorie foods are produced by the replacement of high-calorie nutrients with lower calorie substances, e.g., diet margarine, in which most of the oil is replaced by water (Krieger, 1973).

Another issue for older persons who need to insure an adequate diet relates more to how foods are packaged and marketed. Since so many older persons live alone or as couples, it becomes essential from financial and nutritional perspectives to purchase small quantities. It would appear that for the most part such buying behavior is frustrated. Small quantities, when available, are still priced higher than other sizes (Latchford, 1974).

Watkin (1966) suggests that new lines of food for the aged be formulated in keeping with scientific principles of sound nutrition. It is the opinion of the British scientist, Bender (1971) that there may be considerable advantage in the production of special foods for older persons. Suggestions for characteristics of such "geriatric" foods include: high in necessary nutrients (protein, trace minerals, vitamins), attractive, easy to prepare, acceptable to older persons with attention given to the decline in taste sensation. Bender further notes with surprise that the food industry which has successfully established the "baby foods" has not yet seriously undertaken the profitable marketing of "geriatric foods."

Dietary changes (generally caloric reductions) with age are essential to avoid overweight tendencies and the possibility of obesity. There may be as much as a 600 kcalorie decrease in energy requirements from age 25 to 60. With many middle-aged and older persons, patterns of eating remain almost the same, but activity levels diminish. Fineberg (1972) suggests that "much of the aging process is accelerated by obesity; that it appears safe to say that one of the best ways to stay younger is to maintain normal weight."

MALNUTRITION/UNDERNUTRITION

The final report of the White House Conference on Food, Nutrition and Health (U.S. Government Printing Office, Washington, D.C., 1970) left little doubt that a significant number of older persons in the United States were malnourished. A witness of a Senate Committee in 1970 ventured an educated guess that 8 million of the then 20 million older Americans were malnourished. Soon after, Senator McGovern in an interview, estimated that there are probably more like 10 million who suffer from malnutrition, but are "invisible" since these older persons live in social isolation, many in or near poverty, and are rarely involved in the surveys (GERIATRICS, 1970).

A summary of U.S. dietary surveys of the elderly reveals a high frequency of low calcium and low ascorbic acid intakes suggestive of "inadequate use of milk, fruit and vegetables by the elderly" (Osborn, 1970). Conclusions of researchers who reviewed non-government agency nutritional reports (covering 30,000 subjects, 25 studies, no age specifications) were that the nutritional value of the national diet had fallen noticeably in the period since 1950-55 to 1965 (Davis et al., 1969). Marks, J. (1969) concludes that, based on previous studies in Britain, about 30% of elderly exist in a state of under nutrition while 30% more are close enough to borderline to be easily pushed into undernutrition.

Overnutrition is frequently the focus in the search for life-shortening causes, and only a low level of clinical malnutrition has been observed among older persons due to undernutrition. Nevertheless, clinicians and researchers in the field are more and more convinced there is widespread, if not a growing, subclinical malnutrition among older persons marked by significant nutrient deficiencies (Brink et al., 1968; Corless, 1973; Mayer, 1974; Rao, 1973). Many older persons, during the typical gradual reduction in food intake, cut down on fruits and vegetables, thereby denying themselves essential vitamins and trace minerals as well as the necessary bulk (Agate, 1968; Mayer, 1974).

Physicians see relatively few older persons with frank malnutrition, i.e., the well known deficiency diseases: scurvy, beri beri, and pellagra. Many presenting symptoms of milder malnutrition such as "lack of well being," loss of appetite and body weight, general malaise and listlessness, headache, insomnia and irritability are frequently assumed to be the expected signs of aging or due to non-nutritional causes (Anderson, 1968; Bender, 1971; Clements, 1975; Exton-Smith, 1968 b).

Malnutrition is clearly possible and exists among those with calorie starvation, undernutrition (Pollack, 1967). The existence of a subclinical deficiency, often more than one or two nutrients, frequently signals apathy and a lack of interest in food (Mayer, 1974; Rao, 1973; Taylor, 1973 a,b). This creates a positive feedback condition, exacerbates the malnutrition and leaves the individual older person even more vulnerable, unable to respond appropriately to the stress of infection, injury, or emotional concerns. Chope's (1954) study with 49 persons 50 years or older, which found there were low intakes of vitamin A, niacin, and ascorbic acid four years prior to death, would appear to substantiate the increased vulnerability.

Subclinical malnutrition was found to be prevalent among the elderly of Australia, as demonstrated by nutrition surveys (Silink et al., 1973). A large number of those tested were eating institutional cooked foods, but little raw vegetables, fresh fruit, or fruit juice. Physical well being was related to nutritional status in a study by Kelley et al., (1957) at Michigan State University. The population was made up of 97 white and 104 black women between 40-80 years of age: 95% had nutrient intake below 80% of the RDA for one or more nutrients; 40% described "unexplained tiredness, pains in the joints, and shortness of breath." Those women who had intakes 40% below the RDA for one or more nutrients had a higher mortality rate. It is conceivable, however, that dietary patterns were affected by illness as well as the reciprocal effect (Schlenker et al., 1973). Stress may trigger clinical symptoms of milder malnutrition, or stress may reveal overt malnutrition where no suspicion of subclinical malnutrition existed (Hyams, 1973).

It is also probable that there is a close correlation between the health of older persons and the proportion of dietary energy from protein. Exton-Smith and Stanton (1965) found this to be true. It appears that the primary cell and molecular renewal function of proteins is subverted at times of very low carbohydrate and fat intake. The overall body requirement for energy takes precedence and the protein is thus metabolized to provide energy. Excess protein calories may also be converted to glycogen and stored for future body needs. While controversy over protein require-ments related to age continues, there is increasing evidence that the need for specific amino acids may be greater than considered to date (Theuer, 1971). There may be a critical requirement for high quality proteins, so that the protein-sparing role of carbohydrates may become more significant with advancing age. Supplements of lysine, threonine or proteolytic enzymes have corrected poor nitrogen balance in older persons (Albanese, 1963). Requirements for methi-onine and lysine nearly tripled in one study. The problem of obtaining sufficient amounts of higher quality protein with age is compounded by the decrease in caloric intake (Bigwood, 1966).

REGULATORY SUBSTANCES/GENERAL

Many articles, both in the scientific and lay journals, address the issue of the serious consequences for human nutrition of food processing, particularly the removal of essential micronutrients from grains and sugar. The large losses (20% to 90%) of the micronutrients in refining, processing, canning and cooking of foods may be among the major contributing causes of the poor nutritional status and poor health of many older persons (Schroeder, 1971).

Dr. Henry Schroeder, Director of the Trace Elements Laboratory at Dartmouth Medical School, supplied some of the data to a hearing in Washington, D.C., in August of 1970 (Lear, 1970). He stated that though white bread may contain an adequate number of calories for a healthy diet, it lacks the nutrients that are necessary to use these calories properly in the body. Flour used in the white bread that so many Americans eat is used here only as an example of the kind of "manufactured" deficiencies that exist in many foods. This inadequacy is compounded in older persons, many of whom have a nutritional status already at risk.

Syntheses of DNA and RNA depends on the adequate supply of B_1, B_{12}, and folic acid, but in the processing of flour for white bread, 77% of vitamin B_1 and 67% of folic acid are removed. The vitamins A, D, E, riboflavin, niacin and pyridoxine participate in essential, multiple enzymatic reactions in the human body of any age. Nevertheless, most of vitamin A, 80% of riboflavin, 81% of niacin, 72% of pyridoxine, most of vitamin D and 86% of vitamin E are also removed from the wheat grains (Lear, 1970).

Recent animal and human studies have suggested critical roles for a number of major minerals and trace minerals that are lost in the refining processes of foods (Schroeder, 1971). Forty percent of chromium, 86% of manganese, 16% selenium and 78% of zinc are removed from wheat grains; 76% of the iron, 89% of the cobalt, 60% of the calcium, 78% of the sodium, 77% of the potassium, 85% of the magnesium and 71% of the phosphorus are also found in the residue. Cadmium, a fairly toxic mineral, competes with zinc in human metabolism.

Excess cadmium has been implicated in hypertension, yet its concentration is increased in white flour as compared to whole wheat from 1:20 in white flour as compared with 1:120 in the whole grain product (Schroeder, 1971).

Mineral deficiencies in serum and tissue levels have also received some recent attention. In congestive heart failure, muscle biopsies show evidence of body depletion of magnesium (Lim and Jacobs, 1972). Chromium has been found deficient in persons who have died of heart attacks. Chromium deficiency in animals is characterized by symptoms similar to the degenerative diseases associated with age, such as impaired glucose tolerance, diabetes or cardiovascular disease (Levander, 1975). The addition of zinc to the diet of wounded persons speeds the healing of the wounds (Lear, 1970).

MAJOR MINERALS.

Calcium (Ca). Calcium is the most ubiquitous mineral in the body and may reach between two to three pounds in adults, about 2% of total body weight. The major portion (about 99%) is found in bones and teeth, but about 1% is in muscle and extracellular fluid throughout the body. Calcium in the bone is used by the body as a reservoir (calcium in teeth is less available) from which the mineral may be withdrawn to respond to requirements of cells if dietary Ca is insufficient. Normal serum calcium is 10 milligrams/100ml. Serum levels, quite stable from day to day, are under the primary control of the parathyroid hormone, but also with the participation of the pituitary, adrenal and thyroid hormones. When serum calcium becomes too high, the thyroid hormone, calcitonin, lowers the level of blood calcium by decreasing any mobilization from the bone.

Intestinal absorption of calcium is adequate in most average diets with a phosphate/calcium ratios of 2:1 to 1:1. The absorption rate from the intestine can range from 10-50%. There are other nutrient factors in the diet which may either stimulate or inhibit calcium absorption from the gut. Vitamin D enhances absorption through the intestinal membranes by its involvement in the synthesis of calcium-binding protein. Vitamin C provides the acidic pH which potentiates calcium solubility. In the stomach, the hydrochloric acid environment enables the separation of the calcium ion from food as the digestive breakdown proceeds. Metabolism of any excess fat in the diet will increase the concentration of fatty acids that are likely to interfere with calcium absorption since calcium combines with fatty acids to form insoluble calcium soaps (Stare & McWilliams, 1973). On the other hand, lactose (the sugar in milk) one of the best sources of calcium, can form a soluble complex with calcium and thereby lowers the insoluble complexes that may form, enhancing Ca absorption.

Calcium is essential for optimum ossification of bone and for development of teeth — as calcium phosphates and carbonate (hydroxyapatite crystals). Blood clotting requires calcium to activate blood platelets, in fibrin formations for the clot. Calcium also activates the digestive enzyme pancreatic lipase, in the small intestine, which splits fatty acids from glycerol in nutrient fats. Neuromuscular function also requires calcium for regulating muscle contraction and as a cofactor in the release of the neuro-transmitter acetylcholine. As such, calcium adequacy is essential to avoid irregular tetanic spasms of all muscle, and particularly any irregularities of heart beat. There is considerable concern among physicians and researchers about calcium metabolism, but as with many nutrients, some disagreement exists about its nutritional significance.

The RDA for calcium is 800 milligrams, yet numerous surveys indicate that most of American adults, in particular women homemakers, have a daily intake of only 400 mg. Absorption rate is variable (between 10-50%) and several exit mechanisms exist, e.g., renal excretion (relatively independent of dietary intake), in bile and pancreatic juice and dermal losses. If the amount absorbed from the gut exceeds the calcium loss, calcium will be available for deposition (along with phosphate and fluoride) in bone (Lutwak, 1975). Calcium plays a particularly important role in the nutrition of older persons in the etiology of osteoporosis. Intake of calcium (also potassium and magnesium) for 77 men and 185 women, 65 and over living at home in Glasgow, were reported well below national averages (Macleod et al., 1975). The authors noted the importance of milk and the relevance of calcium to bone disease and aging. Long-term dietary calcium inadequacy has been suggested as a principal cause for osteoporosis (Lutwak, 1964, 1969; Nordin, 1960). Calcium (with fluoride, phosphate and vitamin D) is a critical metabolite in the pathology of osteoporosis.

Further, Nordin (1972) believes that the calcium requirement of post-menopausal women should be increased because of high urinary calcium. Lutwak (1969) notes that intake and ultimate disposition of calcium is interdependent on the metabolism of vitamin D, lipid, phosphate, and fluoride. Animal studies have demonstrated that simple negative calcium balance stimulates the parathyroids and produces resorption of whole bone, leading to osteoporosis. Long term intake of fluoride appears to reduce the incidence of osteoporosis. Hurexthal and Vose (1969) estimated that the total calcium intake in osteoporotics was 21% lower than "normals." Osteoporosis may also result from immobilization (Mack et al., 1967), castration (Davis et al., 1966), and gastrectomy (Morgan et al., 1966).

Periodontal disease is considered by some to be an associated symptom of osteoporosis (Henrikson, 1968). Increased dietary calcium may slow or even reverse the alveolar bone loss and provide a better foundation for the teeth. (Nutrition News, 1970). Calcium supplementation was almost completely absorbed and there was a lasting retention in fluids with calcium provided to 27 subjects (53-89 years) of a nursing home, demonstrating it is relatively simple to compensate for calcium deficiency in older persons.

Potassium (K). Potassium deficiency may represent a very significant problem for older persons. It is essential, with sodium for the electrolytic balance between intracellular and extracellular fluid exchanges. Sodium along with potassium also function in the propagation of the nervous impulse everywhere in the body affecting muscle activities (skeletal and cardiac) as well as intellectual and emotional tasks.

Dietary deficiency of potassium is not normally easily developed. Yet with age, it becomes more widespread. Those individuals who are more vulnerable include persons on restricted diets, those with prolonged diarrhea, kidney dysfunction, diabetic acidosis and diuretic therapy. Potassium depletion is characterized by depressive states, muscle weakness, disorientation, cardiac arrythmias and irritability.

Older persons in their homes have shown a potassium intake lower than the normal younger adult population (Dall and Gardner, 1971). Elderly patients (mean age 75, and 46%

living on their own), with vague symptoms of weakness, inability to concentrate and urinary incontinence were treated with supplementary potassium (Fletcher, 1974): 86% improved in at least one of the symptoms, 63% were less tired, 56% ceased to be depressed, 54% became more able to concentrate, 37% showed improved strength and 19% became continent. Judge and Cowan (1971) found that dietary potassium intake correlates directly with muscle strength, and that it may be an error to assume muscle weakness is a part of physiological aging. Judge (1972) believes that there is extensive subclinical nutritional potassium deficiency easily corrected by nutrition education.

Magnesium (Mg). As a co-factor in cell respiratory reactions involving ATP, magnesium plays an important role in carbohydrate, fat, and protein metabolism as well as the total energy economy of the body. The efficiency of all of these processes is at increasing risk with time.

Magnesium exists in rather small amounts in the soft tissues and skeleton. This ion is found primarily intracellularly with a plasma level of 1.5-1.8 mg. per liter. Approximately 17 of the 25 gms. of magnesium in the adult can be found in bone, the apparent storage site in the body and is mobilized if blood and other tissue levels are depleted. Intake is variable since there is a range of content in different foods (Schroeder, Nason and Tipton, 1969). Absorption from the alimentary tract resembles that of calcium (Judge, 1973). Fifteen to 40 milliequivalents per day is the range for 'healthy' individuals in U.S. and Europe (Seelig, 1964). About the 60-70% of this intake is excreted in the stool (Seelig, 1964) and the rest is lost in sweat, desquamated skin and urine (Wacker, 1964).

Magnesium is involved in protein synthesis, as part of the enzymatic functions in ribosomal aggregation, in binding of messenger RNA to ribosomal particles and in the synthesis and degradation of DNA (Sutherland, 1970). Magnesium is also implicated in neuromuscular transmission, interacting with calcium, either antagonistically or syngeristically (Wacker and Parisi, 1968). In experimental depletion (in 4 recorded studies of small numbers of human volunteers), plasma levels fell to between 10 and 30% of control concentration. Hypocalcemia occurred in 6 of the 7 subjects, in spite of appropriate calcium intake (Shils, 1969) and most exhibited hypokalemia and negative potassium balance. After deficiency periods of from 25-110 days, neurologic signs occurred in 5 of 7 subjects. In addition there was frequent nausea, anorexia and apathy which preceded augmentation of the neurologic changes. Further, Shill (1969) reports that personality changes, spontaneous muscle spasms, tremor and fasciculations developed in the experimentally induced hypomagnesium state. Magnesium deficiency in persons of all ages is rare, since this mineral is found in most vegetables and milk. Yet in a number of complicating disease states, symptomatic human magnesium deficiency can occur — in severe malabsorption, chronic alcoholism/malnutrition, acute or chronic renal disease, excessive use of diuretics, and in surgical patients on parenteral nutrition for a prolonged time (Jones et al., 1969; Randall, 1969; Stare and McWilliams, 1973). It is not difficult to project to a number of situations in which older persons, more prone to the states and conditions listed can and do experience marginal, if not deficient magnesium, and the resulting effects.

TRACE ELEMENTS: Fe, Zn, Se, Ch

Iron (Fe). An optimal nutritional requirement of iron for older persons is difficult to assign. At best, an individual decision would need to be made related to many factors (economics, living style, health and disease).

Normally, body iron is recycled and stored, with no particular mechanism for the excretion of any excess each day. Approximately 8 g. of hemoglobin are synthesized each day to replenish those senescing red blood cells that are broken down. The 26 mg of iron required for the synthesis of new red blood cells is supplied from the released iron of the destroyed erythrocytes. Hemorrhage and menstruation are two means of loss of blood, though not a typical daily occurrence. A regular, very small quantity of iron, an average of 1 milligram, is lost daily in the shedding of cells from the intestinal tract, urinary tissue and the skin (Robertson et al., 1976). Therefore, under relatively normal conditions, only 1 mg of iron must be absorbed from the gut daily. Major control of iron concentration is based in the gut and the iron absorbed is about 10% of the dietary iron. Some balance studies have indicated a mean absorption of 11-14% of dietary iron intake (Jacob and Greenman, 1969). When iron stores are low, absorption may increase two or three times the average 10% – from 1 mg to 3.5 mg daily (Moore, 1965).

There appears to be considerable differences in iron absorption (Callender, 1971) from different foods: e.g. it is more efficient from muscle and hemoglobin than from vegetables and eggs. Iron in brown bread was better absorbed than from iron-enriched bread (in spite of high phytate content). Iron in eggs is poorly absorbed but corrected by orange juice. The fact that egg yolk depresses/inhibits the absorption of iron from other foods is of concern in designing diets.

Zinc (Zn). The average human dietary intake is about 10-15 mg/day of which about 5 mg are retained (Li and Vallee, 1973). Cereals high in phytic acid (which binds zinc and other minerals in the intestine) decrease absorption. In human tissues, the highest concentrations have been reported in the prostate, liver and kidney (Schroeder, et al., 1967) and the total amount has been estimated at between 203 gm.

Low plasma zinc has been found in many chronic diseases, including myocardial infarction (Schroeder, 1971). Human (whole) blood contains about 900 $\mu g/100$ ml; normal serum Zn averages 121 ± 19 $\mu g/100$ ml. Decreased serum zinc has been reported in various malignancies, but no uniform pattern is possible with the available data (Li and Vallee, 1973). Schroeder (1971) also reports that supplements were found to promote wound healing and circulation in ischemic extremities in elderly patients. Soil in many parts of the United States is extremely low in zinc and marginal deficiencies have been known to occur (Robertson, 1976 p. 431). Zinc deficiency may be as common in human physiology as iron and vitamin C deficiencies and appears to be of equal importance, particularly in wound healing (Pullen et al., 1971; Pories et al., 1967). Zinc may be involved in atherosclerosis since high Zn/Cu ratios have been found in hypocholesterolemic patients (Klevay, 1975).

A reduction in taste acuity may be one of the symptoms of zinc deficiency which may also be accompanied by a reduction in the capacity for smell as well. With the effect upon these two senses so involved with the response to attractiveness of food, appetite already diminished in older persons may be further decreased. This may be especially true of those persons who use an increased quantity of processed or "convenience" foods.

Selenium (Se). Selenium is a trace mineral essential to plants and animals including the human being, but toxic at certain levels. It appears to be involved with vitamin E metabolism as a catalyst in electron transport. Information about selenium metabolism is fragmentary (Li and Vallee, 1973). Selenium, and selenium containing amino acids similar to vitamin E, inhibit lipid peroxidation, breakdown free radicals and so can protect against radiation damage. It is conceivable then that selenium and selenium containing amino acids may participate in the stability of biologic membrances of mitochondria, microsomes and lysosomes. It is unlikely that human selenium deficiency exists except in extremely malnourished individuals. However, it is noted here because of its frequent linkage with vitamin E.

Chromium (Ch). Chromium, present in minute amounts in blood and various tissues, is in high concentration at birth and declines with age. A particular role for chromium has been identified in carbohydrate and lipid metabolism of animals and specifically glucose utilization. It has been suggested that chromium facilitates the binding of insulin to cell membranes (Mertz, 1967). Supplementation with chromium for maturity-onset diabetics has improved glucose tolerance (Glinsman and Mertz, 1966; Levine, et al., 1968; Schroeder, 1971).

Chromium levels have been reported as low in the American population. Chronic chromium deficiency has been implicated in hypercholesterolemia, glucose intolerance, and lipid deposition in the aorta (Schroeder, 1971). The interrelationship appears reasonable. Chromium levels decline with age, and the last two conditions mentioned increase with the years. Schroeder notes further that chromium supplements have also been used with some success to treat older persons with hypercholesterolemia.

VITAMINS: DEFICIENCIES AND FUNCTIONS

Vitamins are intimately involved in metabolic pathways as co-enzymes in hundreds of enzymatic reactions. A deficiency of even one vitamin may therefore have consequences for many divergent functions and various tissues. There is still uncertainty related to vitamin requirements in the last half of life. Inadequate information about changes in absorption capacity, the significance of subclinical or marginal vitamin malnutrition and the multiple interactions of nutrition with the psychological, social, and economic realities of older persons accounts for the lack of definite statements.

The use of a variety of biochemical and modified clinical tests relevant to vitamin status is not always appreciated. In older persons, existing body reserves of vitamins may be diminished below critical levels before typical overt clinical symptoms are observed. Biochemical clues frequently precede clinical malnutrition: the decrease in vitamin C concentration in leucocytes, low serum folate levels, or changes in serum alkaline phosphatase reflective of vitamin D deficiency and osteomalacia.

FAT-SOLUBLE VITAMINS

Vitamins A, D, E, and K are normally broken down into micelles and absorbed in the intestine in the presence of bile salts. Hyper-vitaminosis A and D have been demonstrated, suggesting therefore that a storage capacity for vitamins may have both advantages and disadvantages.

Vitamin A. Low intakes of vitamin A, niacin, and ascorbic acid were observed four years prior to death among 49 individuals 50 years or older studied by Chope (1954). Low vitamin A was correlated with the heightened incidence of nervous, circulatory and respiratory diseases. It is also possible that malabsorption of vitamin A may result in chronic lesions, e.g., eye lesions and follicular hyperkeratosis (Kirk and Chieffi, 1952) which improved with administration of the vitamin. Significantly, these lesions are frequent in older persons and have been accepted as "normal" concomitants of aging. These so-called "normal" changes may indeed by the observable signs of subclinical malnutrition.

Vitamin D. Vitamin D_2 is produced by irradiating the provitamin ergosterol in plants and vitamin D_3 is produced by the irradiation of the provitamin 7 dehydrocholesterol found underneath the skin.

There is little in the literature related to vitamin D metabolism of the adult and even less related to the older person. However, there is some indication that older patients who have long stays in the hospital and house-bound persons may indeed have inadequate dietary vitamin D (Baker, 1962; Corless et al., 1973; Exton-Smith and Stanton, 1965; Macleod et al., 1974). Further, it is reasonable to question the dietary adequacy of those older persons who have little or no milk (or milk products) in their diets and who do not have (or take advantage of) the opportunity for exposure to sunlight. Smith, et al., (1964) suggest a causal, inverse relationship between exposure to sunlight and involutional osteoporosis. Any pathology which interferes with absorption of vitamin D, calcium and phosphorus may result in osteomalacia.

Vitamin E, tocopherols and tocotrienols. Alpha-tocopherol is the most biologically active of the series of vitamin E compounds called tocopherols and tocotrienols. Vitamin E, a group of closely related substances is present in leafy vegetables, whole grains and vegetable oils. As with the aforementioned two fat soluble vitamins A and D, vitamin E is stored in the body. Early work done over 40 years ago dealt primarily with vitamin E deficiencies in non-human animals: heart damage in calves; muscular dystrophy in chicks; rabbits and guinea pigs; liver degeneration, growth retardation and reproductive failure in rats. However, in humans with similar ailments, massive doses of vitamin E have had no measurable benefit (FDA Consumer, July/Aug., 1973).

Watkin (1973) reports some work from Canada which indicates a role for vitamin E in protein synthesis. Contrary to extravagant claims related to large doses there is some evidence that increased ingestion of vitamin E leads to decreased absorption (Witting, 1975). Although it is a relatively poor antioxidant, vitamin E is expected to limit, if not completely inhibit the rate of synthesis of the damaging free radicals in body tissues (Witting, 1975). Studies have demonstrated that the vitamin does minimize the peroxidative damage to subcellular membranes (Witting, 1975).

The widely accepted correlation of dietary saturated fats and atherosclerosis has increased the dietary intake of polyunsaturates. This degree of unsaturation increases the need for tocopherols. Extrapolating from the kinetics of autoxidation *in vitro*, it is unlikely that "massive ingestion of vitamin E" would have an appreciable effect on aging processes. It is conceivable with the current use of polyunsaturated fats, that a vitamin E deficiency disease may develop. Even frank deficiency does not produce clear-cut symptoms. However, it has been suggested that as the polyunsaturated fats in diets increase, so does the vitamin E content (Bieri, 1976), since most sources of polyunsaturated fats also contain vitamin E.

Not all deficiencies are dietary. Herting (1967) reports patients that suffer with malabsorptive disorders are characterized by a number of classic symptoms of vitamin E deficiency. The Food and Nutrition Board's RDA (1974) indicates the requirement for vitamin E for adults is in a range between 10-15 international units (I.U.). Herting disagrees with this adult tocopherol requirement. In view of the facts that relatively normal populations have demonstrated vitamin E deficiency and that the content of vitamin E in many foods is low, he suggests that it is important to insure optimum vitamin E ingestion (and levels). This is especially significant for those who may be ill or malnourished as well as for the "healthy" individuals who have unkowingly limited their intake (Herting, 1967; Watkin, 1973).

Vitamin K. Vitamin K prevents hemorrhaging. It participates indirectly in the blood-clotting mechanism by affecting the concentration of other factors — prothrombin, proconvertin, and thromboplastin in the plasma. Deficiency of vitamin K delays blood-clotting time. A dietary deficiency in adults is rare because vitamin K is found in most leafy plants and is also synthesized by intestinal bacteria.

In the presence of any one or more conditions such as liver dysfunction, biliary disorder, antibiotic therapy, prolonged salicylate use, uremia, mineral oil ingestion and inadequate intestinal absorption, a deficiency may be precipitated. Unfortunately, there is a high percentage of these disorders in a large number of elderly persons. A study completed on a random sample of 110 patients admitted to a hospital in Essex, age range 56-100 years, found 75% of those persons with a low thrombotest (for vitamin K). With oral vitamin K therapy there was a fairly quick return to normal. In some, the etiology of this deficiency was clear; hepatic damage or anticoagulant drugs; in others, etiology was unknown (Hazell and Baloch, 1970).

THE WATER-SOLUBLE VITAMINS

The water-soluble vitamins include a group of unlike substances present in many of the same foods. For a variety of reasons, the foods which contain these vitamins are eaten in decreased amounts by people in the last half of life; fresh fruits and vegetables, whole-grain cereals, some meats, eggs and milk. Unlike fat-soluble vitamins, there is very little storage of water-soluble vitamins and the small pool that is maintained, is related to the saturation capacity of an apoenzyme. In early, mild malnutrition of any one of the B-complex vitamins, the symptomology is similar. Only advanced deficiencies produce clearly different manifestations for each of the vitamins. Some geriatricians have found that therapeutic doses of water-soluble vitamins may be needed to correct long-standing vitamin deficiencies found in large numbers of older people (Fleck, 1976). The vitamin B-complex represents a group of vitamins, chemically different, yet generally bound together in nature, which function similarly.

Thiamin, Vitamin B_1. Thiamin is one of the vitamins in which older persons are likely to be deficient. Currently, the RDA for the over 51 group is 1.2 mg for males and 1.0 mg for females (Food and Nutrition Board 1974). Many of the foods less frequently used in the diet mentioned earlier are excellent sources of vitamin B_1. Deficiency of this vitamin may be due to possible difficulty with chewing and probable difficulty with the high cost of aforementioned food. Brin et al., (1964) reported the average thiamin intake of 0.7 mg for elderly men in a community home for the aged in Syracuse, N.Y.

In a number of older persons, there may be an inactivation of thiamine, due largely to gastric achlorhydria and altered intestinal flora which bind ingested thiamin (Whanger, 1973). Thus, a deficiency develops due not to age *per se* but to a disorder accompanying age.

A necessary participant in the pentose phosphate metabolism is thiamin pyrophosphate (TPP) coenzyme for erythrocytic transketolase. Brin, et al., (1964), found that more than 10% of the elderly living at home were provided with inadequate dietary amounts of ascorbic acid, thiamine and riboflavin. Daily intake is even more important than with fat-soluble vitamins since stores of thiamin (and other B vitamins) are depleted very quickly.

As with a number of other nutrients, requirements are variable in response to particular conditions. Requirements increase during fever, elevated carbohydrate intake, malignancy, and the increased excretion of thiamin with diuretic therapy. It is fact that many older persons are more susceptible to these dysfunctions and experience them with greater frequency than younger persons.

Cheraskin et al., (1967) note greater frequency of cardiovascular complaints in older persons who ingest small quantities of thiamin. Schlenker, et al., (1973) reexamined a group of women originally studied in 1948 to 1955. One of the nutrients, thiamin, appeared to be related to cardiovascular accidents. Women who had high dietary thiamin had a lower incidence of death from cardiovascular disease.

Riboflavin, Vitamin B_2. This vitamin functions as the prosthetic group of the active flavoprotein enzymes. These enzymes are involved in electron transport and are participants in a number of oxidative enzymes systems.

Generally, riboflavin deficiency occurs only in conjunction with other B-complex deficiencies. The symptomology frequently associated with riboflavin deficiency: glossitis, cheilosis, and seborrheic dermatitis of the nose and scrotum may also relate to more widespread deficiencies. Rivlin (1970) has reivewed the possible relationship between riboflavin deficiencies and hormone imbalances. Cellular growth cannot prosper in the absence of riboflavin, since a primary energy-producing group of enzymatic reactions would be severely slowed or inhibited.

The need for riboflavin is increased during tissue repair (wound healing) consequent to surgery, burns, or trauma, and generally during growth (protein synthesis), more specifically as a result of testosterone propionate therapy. As a matter of fact, the increased need for riboflavin and protein go hand in hand. Older persons are obviously at greater risk in meeting these conditions satisfactorily, and have been shown to be deficient in both thiamin and riboflavin in the American survey studies of Brin (1968) and Dibble et al., (1967). Similar information came from the Netherlands Institute of Nutrition, Amsterdam, which reported that old people had a higher incidence of low and insufficient intake of vitamins A, ascorbic acid, thiamin and riboflavin that the younger group (Dalderup et al., 1970). Low thiamin intake of older people was associated with diseases of the nervous and circulatory systems (Schlenker et al., 1973).

Pyridoxine, Vitamin B_6. Vitamin B_6 occurs in a wide range of foods: meats, cereals, lentils, nuts and vegetables. As a coenzyme, it is involved in a large number of different enzymatic systems (as many as 60) related primarily to nitrogen metabolism. Noteworthy also is its role with phosphorylase, the enzyme that catalyzes the breakdown of glycogen to glucose $- 1 -$ phosphate.

Deficiency in human adults was first reported in 1939 (Spies et al.,) with symptoms of weakness, irritability, nervousness, insomnia, and difficulty in walking. Marked decrease and disappearance of symptoms were achieved within 24 hours of pyridoxine administration. It was also reported effective with cheilosis not responsive to riboflavin therapy (Smith and Martin, 1940).

Very few reports appear in the literature relating to vitamin B_6 deficiency among older persons. However, mention has been made of an increase in requirement with hyperthyroidism and with increased protein ingestion.

Niacin, Vitamin B_3. NAD (DPN), nicotinamide adenine dinucleotide and NADP (TPN), nicotinamide adenine dinucleotide phosphate, are coenzymes which function as hydrogen and electron acceptors, participants in cellular respiration and in carbohydrate, fat, and protein metabolism. Niacin may be synthesized in the body from the dietary amino acid, tryptophan (Horwitt, 1955).

Levels if niacin (in addition to vitamins A and C) were low for four years before death in 49 persons 50 years or older in the study by Chope (1954). Whanger (1973) reports that niacin tissue levels are "somewhat decreased in elderly persons." Pellagra, the disease syndrome which results from significant and frank niacin deficiency, is rarely seen today. Among older persons, the concern is with the subclinical deficiency of niacin. Found (along with other B-complex vitamins) in legumes, liver, meats and yeast, it is conceivable that older persons who are alcoholics, food faddists, or who suffer malabsorptive disorders would be in a niacin deficient state though not exhibiting the dermatitis, diarrhea and dementia typical of pellagra.

More important may be the relationship of niacin to blood levels of lipids. Large doses of nicotinic acid (from 3-6 g /day) appears to lower the levels of cholesterol, beta-lipoproteins and the glycerides in the blood (Miller, et al., 1960; Shawyer, et al., 1961). The suggested roles for lipids and cholesterol in the etiology of atherosclerosis and cardiovascular dysfunction could give significance to a niacin deficiency among older persons.

Folacin. Folacin includes folic acid and related compounds. As a coenzyme it has a central role in single carbon metabolism, and functions in purine and pyrimidine synthesis (the bases in nucleic acid structure). Folacin is bound to protein, often conjugated and absorbed easily from the gastrointestinal tract. In conjunction with vitamin B_{12} and ascorbic acid, folacin is necessary for red blood cell synthesis. Under "normal" conditions, total body folate stores are between 5-10 mg.

Nutritional deficiency of folacin (as well as regulatory nutrients and protein) may be the result of at least one or more of these five steps: inadequate ingestion (dietary), absorption, and utilization; increased requirement and increased excretion (Herbert, 1973). At each of these steps, there are conditions of existence of the last half of life that could lead to folate deficiency.

inadequate ingestion: any chronic disorder of the upper one-third of the small intestine and/or drugs such as dilantin, barbiturates may lead to inadequate absorption.

inadequate utilization: may be involved with a metabolic block such as an enzyme deficiency liver disease, vitamins B_{12} and C deficiencies.

increased requirement: chronic blood loss, hyperthyroidism or malignancy could create an increased requirement for folacin.

In the BRITISH MEDICAL JOURNAL, F. Murphy et al., (1969) reported investigations done on 1,004 new patients over 50 years of age who were admitted to mental hospitals. They stated that, "dementia due to folate deficiency should be considered if an elderly mental patient has a history suggestive of nutritional deficiency." In these individuals, there may be the early subclinical signs of lassitude, apathy and weakness. Vitamin C deficiency may also exist. In another study there was a significant correlation between low serum folate and organic brain disease (Batata et al., 1967). While megaloblastic anemia, directly tied to folacin deficiency, is not common in older persons, folate reserves are low in older persons (Exton-Smith, 1968 b).

The possibility of neuropathy as a sequel to subclinical deficiencies concerns the gerontologist. It is noteworthy that two cases of severe dementia apparently due to folate deficiency responded with complete recovery with folic acid treatment. Strachan et al., (1967) found low folic acid levels in 80% of the old persons waiting to get into British Welfare homes. In many folacin-deficient persons glossitis, diarrhea, and even megaloblastic anemia are observable.

Cobalamin, Vitamin B_{12}. Cobalamin is the antipernicious anemia factor and found almost exclusively in animal tissues — liver, kidney, oysters. It is synthesized by some intestinal flora, and functions as coenzyme to stimulate red blood cell formation, in the synthesis of nucleic acid and nucleoprotein, and in the metabolic pathways of nervous tissue.

Pernicious anemia is the classic deficiency state but is not a major problem for the majority of older persons. Of greater significance is the relationship of the subclinical deficiencies of folacin and vitamin B_{12} which may be involved with confusion and psychiatric disorders (Kallstrom and Nylof, 1969).

Inadequate, poorly planned vegetarian diets (frequently those which omit any and all animal products) and impaired absorption affect the store and availability of vitamin B_{12}. Pathology such as abnormal protein synthesis, liver or renal disease, malignancy of the intestine may interfere seriously with adequate absorption. In one report from Israel (Abramsky, 1972), data of three elderly patients with neurological manifestations of vitamin B_{12} deficiency (no anemia) are discussed. Several months after the initiation of treatment with cyanocabalamin, the patients were almost cured. Vitamin B_{12} was administered to elderly persons, 65 to 90 years old who complained of fatigue. The symptoms disappeared for 89% of the cases. When the vitamin was replaced with a placebo, the symptoms reappeared (Fleck, 1976).

Although levels of serum vitamin B_{12} vary a great deal in older persons, there have been sufficient reports in the literature to warrant the conclusion that vitamin B_{12} deficiency (along with folacin deficiency) are known causes of dementia and confusional states (Mitra, 1970).

Ascorbic acid, Vitamin C. Ascorbic acid, a most unstable vitamin, is recommended at a level of 45 mg daily. It contributes to normal functioning of all cells, including subcellular structures and is essential for the formation of normal collagen. Vitamin C is a coenzyme involved in the conversion of folic acid to the active folinic acid. It may also be important in the body utilization of vitamin B_{12}. Vitamin C facilitates the absorption of iron from the intestine, participates in detoxification processes, and maintains the integrity of blood vessels. It is a powerful antioxidant and is considered important in the protection of other antioxidants, vitamin E, polyunsaturates, fatty acids and vitamin A. Conflicting evidence mounts here and there is need for further research.

Vitamin C may act through the adrenals on protein metabolism (Eckhardt and Davidson, 1948). ACTH (pituitary trophic hormone), in sufficient amounts, quickly exhausts the cells of the adrenal cortex of their cholesterol and vitamin C stores. Response to stress involves this sequelae and repeated daily stress is part of the life style of many middle-aged and older persons. Cholesterol metabolism was thought to be responsive to ascorbic acid, though the mechanism was unknown (Bronte-Stewart et al., 1963). For a number of years, Russian physicians prescribed a high intake of vitamin C to inhibit hypercholesterolemia, thereby preventing atherosclerosis (Simonson and Keys, 1961).

In a longitudinal study of 100 women whose dietary records date back to 1948, Schlenker (1973) found (as did Chope in 1954) that there was a relationship between mortality and vitamin C intake. Sixty women had died between 1948 and 1972 and had lower vitamin C and protein intake than those who survived (in 1948 and 1972). Most American investigators have been unable to confirm these observations.

Atherosclerosis has been produced in animals by inducing vitamin C deficiency though the serum level of cholesterol was normal (Willis, 1953). Recently, Stamler (1970) reported that "the mortality rates for middle-aged persons with hypertensive disease and stroke have dropped significantly, due in part to improved nutritional management, including adequate intake of vitamin C (Riccitelli, 1972). Dr. Spittle in LANCET (1971, 1972) reports that older people have lower levels of vitamin C than younger persons. Further, she adds, "atherosclerosis is a long-term deficiency of vitamin C that permits cholesterol to build up in the arterial system." Subclinical deficiency of vitamin C may be manifest by gum swelling and hemorrhage of nasal, intestinal, menstrual, sublingual tissues and skin (Chazan et al., 1963; Taylor, 1974, 1975). Mitra (1969) presented very interesting case histories of vitamin C deficiency in the elderly related to multiple bruises, malignancy, leg pain, etc. Elderly men have lower levels of ascorbic acid than older women (Morgan et al., 1955). Inadequate diet and malabsorption were cited by Anderson (1968) as important in the frequent deficiencies observed in the elderly, especially of vitamin C and folacin. The lead article in BRITISH MEDICAL JOURNAL, 13 September, 1969, suggests that an elderly patient with mental symptoms be checked for deficiencies of folacin, B_{12}, potassium and vitamin C (referred to in folacin discussion earlier in this report).

Vitamin C has been suggested as an important factor in

resistance to respiratory disease by Cheraskin et al., (1973) since its introduction is able to reduce the appearance of respiratory symptomology. Regnier (1968) and others (Wilson, 1974) have reported favorable results with administration of large doses of vitamin C in prevention and treatment of the common cold. There are continued investigations into the efficacy of vitamin C preventive and treatment therapy for colds. Many clinicians and researchers remain ambivalent, some dismiss its use, having found no significant effect in short term studies. In a controlled study of two year duration that provided vitamin C supplementation to 297 elderly people (with low blood levels) living in the community, vitamin C "produced no apparent benefits in terms of mortality, morbidity or mental senescence" in spite of measurable increases in plasma and leucocyte vitamin C levels (Burr et al., 1975). However, the same investigators followed all of the group screened for the study (828 elderly persons) and found there was a higher mortality rate among those with low leucocyte ascorbic acid levels (below 15 mg/10^8) than among the remainder. Further, they were able to conclude that the effect was not due to smoking, but more likely to either decreased appetite or effect of illness/disease on plasma levels of vitamin C.

In response to the Burr et al., (1975) statement of 'no apparent benefit of vitamin C supplementation,' Bermond (1976) reports that the results of three trials (two in France, the third in Switzerland), support the evidence that low plasma ascorbic acid is associated with a higher morbidity (symptoms recorded) and with age.

There has been little agreement as well, in the literature on the role of vitamin C in aging processes, changes in tissue repair, collagen metabolism and arteriosclerosis. Yet those conditions that cause acute and chronic stress, and are accompanied by increased liberation of ACTH (adrenocorticotropin hormone), drain the vitamin C available in the adrenals. In severe stress, following serious illness, fractures or surgery, requirements for B-complex and ascorbic acid are notably increased (Riccitelli, 1972). During convalescence increased dosage would seem reasonable and recommended.

SUMMARY

Controversy continues so that more definitive studies with adequate controls are required that could answer questions about efficacy and/or toxicity. Countless reports have now accumulated related to low blood or tissue levels of the water soluble vitamins in older persons:

thiamin: Brin et al., 1964; Brin et al., 1965; Griffiths et al., 1967.

folic acid: Read et al., 1965; Hurdle and Williams, 1966; Batata et al., 1967; Girdwood et al., 1967.

vitamin B_{12}: Hyams, 1964; Dept. of Health and Social Security (Britain), 1972.

vitamin C: Kataria et al., 1965; Andrews and Brook, 1966; Griffiths et al., 1967; Brook and Scrimshaw, 1968; Milne et al., 1971.

Environmental conditions and/or situations of living of many older persons that may contribute to an inadequate diet (and particularly in relation to vitamins) include:

1. poor dentition, which frequently leads to elimination of salads and meats,
2. inability or reluctance to shop for a variety of foods, related to transportation and income,
3. Loss of partner (death or divorce) contributes to the lack of motivation to cook a balanced meal, leads to overuse of refined carbohydrates and sugar-rich beverages, and
4. institutional and/or restaurant cooking provide meals with significant loss of heat-labile vitamins.
5. stress of various kinds.

While it is not clear that lowered levels of vitamins, major minerals and trace elements indicated in these studies are in fact abnormal, there is strong evidence for that suggestion. Particularly persuasive are the results of supplementation with each of the substances which has generally raised the concentrations to "normal" (Hyams, 1973).

OTHER REGULATORY SUBSTANCES

Water. One of the most significant changes with age is in the capacity to maintain homeostatis . . . to sustain a relative constancy of the body's internal environment. Water, considered by many nutritionists as one of the more essential nutrients, is an active substance in this complicated mechanism. Other regulatory materials which contribute to this activity include sodium, potassium, chloride, calcium, magnesium, sulfate, hydrogen ion and phosphorus (Vander et al., 1975). Most of these are in ample supply within an adequate diet.

Without water, survival of the human being is considered limited to four days (Labuza, 1975). All metabolic reactions in the body occur in an aqueous medium and even small changes in tissue and fluid content can interfere with normal metabolism. The composition, concentration and volume of body fluids, with water as a base, is dependent upon the appropriate body monitoring of the electrolyte and fluid balance.

Body water percentage varies with age and body fat, from 50 to 75 percent, and is maintained by way of daily losses through the lungs, kidneys, bowels and skin and daily intake through ingestion. Body water includes tissue water, water from oxidative metabolism and ingested water from food and fluid intake.

Water is within the outside of all cells, part of the constant interchange of intracellular and extracellular fluids for the regulation of osmotic pressure and the exchange of nutrients and gases (Burton, 1976). Water also functions in the regulation of body temperature, in digestive and synthetic processes, as a medium for the disposal of wastes and as a lubricant in all parts of the body (Robinson, 1972). Varying with geographical areas, water could contribute significantly to trace element needs for fluoride, copper and zinc (Guthrie, 1975).

As a medium solvent for all digestive processes, water is of critical importance from point of entry (mouth) to point of exit (anus). Starting with the saliva, water aids in the conversion of daily food to assimilable units. Liquefying of food during the chewing process initiates the digestive conversion and the normal movement of ingested food through the alimentary canal. In addition, the gastric glands, liver, pancreas and intestinal glands produce liquids (with digestive enzymes) which process food in the digestive tract. All along the way, the bolus must be properly liquefied to aid peristalsis, and finally defecation.

Normally, liquid intake should be sufficient to produce a quart or more of urine per day. Each day, the adult loses an average of 2550 milliliters of water (Vander et al., 1975). These losses are generally exactly replaced as a result of a highly integrated group of processes, some controlled, others less so. The sensation called "thirst," by far the most important, is under the integrative, feedback control of the hypothalamus (Whitney and Hamilton, 1977). Urinary loss represents the single largest volume of water removed from the body and is also under a complicated control mechanism involving hormones, neuronal receptors and the hypothalamus.

The literature (to be cited in later chapters on gastrointestinal function and pathology) refers to constipation and urinary dysfunction in older persons. Restriction of fluids, which appears to be a fairly common practice among the aged, may exacerbate both disorders.

The importance of water balance can be viewed from another perspective. With age, there is a change in the distribution of water. Total body water highest at birth diminishes to approximately 50% by age 60 (Guthrie, 1975). The greater loss appears to be in the intracellular volume.

Simple dehydration is the most frequent disturbance observed in the elderly — and effects both electrolyte as well as fluid balance. If deprivation of water (in fluid and solid food intake) is continuous and severe, metabolic processes of synthesis and catabolism are so seriously altered that critical mineral, vitamin and protein deficiencies (explained in greater detail elsewhere in this monograph) may result, which in turn mimic the symptoms of "chronic brain syndrome" — . . . apathy, mental confusion, paranoid behavior, depression, dysphagia, withdrawal, even coma.

Quite another picture can develop with retention of sodium and water found in congestive cardiac failure, hypoproteinemia increased venous pressure, primary renal disease and iatrongenically from the use of corticosteroids, androgens, estrogens and anabolic steroids (Brocklehurst, 1973).

If water is not in balance, the ions (sodium, potassium, manganese) are also affected, and may result in frequently observed lassitude and body weakness. What has been assumed to be an inevitable "mark of age" may then be due to an electrolyte/fluid imbalance, subject to prevention and/or control.

Fiber. "There is no direct evidence that lack of dietary fiber actually causes any disease" . . . But there are statistical correlations between a "fiber-depleted diet and increased incidence" (Weininger and Briggs, 1976).

It has been estimated that 30-40% of the population over 60 in Great Britain have diverticulosis — but only 10% of these individuals have symptoms. There is no adequate survey of the prevalance of diverticulosis in the United States but it is "probable that disability from this cause affects between 5% and 10% of those over 60 years" (Almy, 1976).

The data support for the connection between a whole host of different diseases and fiber (among them — diverticular disease, ulcerative colitis, gallstones, ischemic heart disease, diabetes, obesity, dental caries, etc.) are largely epidemiologic. This evidence indicates a low incidence of these diseases in developing societies and a much higher incidence in affluent, developed societies. There is some difficulty with epidemiologic studies since such data cannot easily identify the causal factors, "changes in the consumption of meat, fat, fiber, sugar, etc. appear to occur simultaneously everywhere" (Hegsted, 1977). In non-human animals, controlled feeding studies could identify long-term, lifetime effects of a range of dietary nutrients. Unfortunately, no such 'feeding' investigations over major portions of the life span are possible with humans.

There are alimentary functions that are clearly affected by dietary fiber, e.g., "the ability of vegetable dietary fiber to increase stool weight" (Eastwood, 1977). The effectiveness of dietary fiber in this task varies, related to the water holding capacity of the fiber and to the amount of fiber in the plants. Different plant sources demonstrate a range of efficiency, e.g., 200g of water can be held by 55g of bran, 100g of raw carrot, 150g of apple and 200g of orange (Eastwood, 1977).

Different vegetable fibers appear to affect serum cholesterol concentration, in a variety of complex action, probably related to the diverse origins and chemistry of the fiber. Some may bring about an increase in the excretion of faecal bile acid, by adsorption or by increasing the movement of faeces (Eastwood, 1977). Unquestionably, different components in 'dietary fibers' produce a variety of metabolic effects on the intestinal contents. However, generalizations about particular effects of 'dietary fibers' do not provide sufficient information for etiological or therapeutic purposes.

Trowell's (1972) hypothesis that dietary fiber may play a protective role in coronary heart disease implicated wheat fiber, which was already identified with an effect on colonic function. But, recent rat experiments (Ranhotra, 1973; Tsai et al., 1976) found plasma cholesterol unaffected when up to 20% bran was added to the diet compared with controls (no added fiber) or when whole wheat flour was compared with white flour at 65% of the diet (Kay and Truswell, 1975). In human studies, the wheat fiber picture is even less definitive, but a number of different investigators conclude there "is not substantial reduction of plasma lipids in short term experiments" (Truswell, 1977). There are, however, increasing reports on the effectiveness of pectin (another fiber) in the significant reduction of plasma cholesterol.

Arguments concerning the importance of dietary fiber come from empirical treatment studies rather than controlled experimental investigations. The use of bran as treatment in constipation, diverticular disease and the spasticity of an irritable bowel (recognized by the small, pellety stool) results in an apparently high rate of recovery. It is noteworthy that up to very recent years, the treatment of choice was the removal of fiber from the diet to ameliorate diverticular and general bowel disease. The work of Neil Painter (Painter and Burkitt, 1971), Hugh Trowell (1960, 1973) and Dennis Burkitt (1973) have been the basis of the improved successful therapy for such patients, many of whom are older.

Most recently, there is mention that too much 'dietary fiber' may result in possible non-absorption or reduced absorption of nutrients as a result of 'too fast' passage through the gastrointestinal tract. Levin (1977) cautions against unqualified statements concerning the "advantages of increased fiber in the diet." His caution grows from several research studies which he states demonstrated that large amounts of dietary fiber decrease serum levels of Mg, Zn, Ca and Fe.

A conference reported in *NUTRITION REVIEWS* (March 1977) concluded, that in view of the still incomplete assessment of the nature of 'dietary fiber' and the varied effectiveness of a variety of fiber containing foods, "that a variety of foods be included in the diet so as to assure the consumption of good mixtures of plant fibers." The challenge remains to identify more carefully and specifically the effects of a variety of dietary residues from fruit, vegetable and whole grain cereal sources. This would require analytic procedures not yet in use (White, Dahlqvist, Pilnek and Trowell, 1977).

Functional Changes: Digestive, Metabolic 4

GASTROINTESTINAL CHANGES

In spite of the apparently widespread gastrointestinal ailments and complaints among the older population, it would appear that the "anatomical and physiological integrity of the gastrointestinal tract" remains at a more than a satisfactory level (Berman and Kirsener, 1972a). There have been mistaken notions about the incidence of life-threatening and disabling disorders of the "aging gut." However, there are some functional changes with age, as well as increasing incidence of malignancy of the large intestine.

Some changes that are involved with time may include altered mobility of the esophagus, lowered acid secretion of the stomach or possibly gastric atrophy. More frequently, digestive disorders in this area are related to other dysfunctions that affect the general well-being, physically and emotionally. Drug abuse among the elderly (induced by physicians as well as older persons themselves) has no doubt contributed to the marked increase of iatrogenic disorders, e.g., the misuse of salicylates, laxatives and strong sedatives.

The most frequent disorders include constipation, diverticulosis, polyps, and cancer. Additional important pathologies include hiatus hernia (esophagus) gastric ulcer, ulcerative colitis, viral hepatitis and cholelithiasis.

DIGESTIVE CAPACITY

It is generally thought there is more frequent abdominal distress with age. There may be some functional changes with time that interfere with the total digestive process, absorption or excretion of nutrients. Malnutrition may also contribute to gastrointestinal dysfunction, e.g. protein deficiency may damage the intestinal mucosa, niacin deficiency may result in diarrhea and riboflavin deficiency brings about cheilosis and some changes in the tongue (Balsley et al., 1971).

One study of 26 subjects (1 woman and 25 men) aged 60-75, in normal health and without digestive complaints provided the following information:

1. With age, digestive gastric secretion is slightly reduced in volume and is less acid.

2. Secretory power of the stomach is somewhat reduced (particularly HC1).

3. Pepsin activity is reduced by one-third.

4. Supplemental digestive enzymes may be advisable in some cases to avoid subclinical deficiencies.

A survey of 3 age groups, 724 pensioners 67 or more, 270 middle-aged people and 180 persons aged 20-24 found (Werner and Hambracus, 1972):

1. In the young group there is little or no complaint, but there are complaints about abdominal distress and constipation in one-third of the elderly group.

2. Food intolerance is rare among the young and fairly common among the old.

3. Fat intolerance is prevalent in about 10% of the older persons, but is essentially absent in the young.

4. There is little or no difference between the middle-aged and older group. This suggests that the primary changes occur before the age of 50, and therefore are not

characteristic of old age.

5. In a group of 8 patients, 67-72 years of age, of good nutritional status and no gastrointestinal complaints, experiments with different levels of fat and protein were carried out to expose any marginal digestive insufficiency. The effects of both a high fat and high protein load proved to result in the excretion of abnormally large amounts of fat and fecal N respectively among the older persons as compared to the younger control group.

6. The high fat diet was handled well when it was divided over all the meals per day. But if 50% of fat was consumed in one meal, digestive insufficiency was noticeable in the increased fecal N. These results suggest a lessened capacity to digest fat, a decreased facility in the utilization of the ingested protein, and that meal size was a determinant in fat tolerance.

Possible explanations for digestive inefficiency with age may include vascular disturbances and degenerative changes of digestive glands which could lead to reduction in protein synthesis (digestive enzymes) and absorption from the gut.

Clearly, the mechanisms for digestive disturbance need quantitative study to determine their significance for nutritional status and health of the older person. Little information is available but a few facts have emerged: parietal cells of the stomach diminish in their capacity for HC1 secretion, there is a reduction in secretion of digestive juices, a decrease in calcium absorption, a decrease in the motility of the gastrointestinal tract, a reduction in blood flow and an overall reduction in the responsiveness and speed of the neurons of the autonomic nervous system that innervate the digestive tract. It is the nervous system that makes the significant connection between the affect and psyche of the older person and digestion. The changes and particular stresses that face older persons more than any other age group create the substrate for biochemical insult and injury to the functional tissues of the digestive system.

Esophagus. Incidence of esophageal hiatus hernia under 40 years is 9% as compared with 60% among the 70+ (Pridie, 1966). Etiology is not always clear but is most frequently assigned to muscle weakness, straining at stool or wearing constricting clothes. In general, hiatus hernias are asymptomatic, but some "complications may include esophagitis, esophageal stricture, bleeding and ulceration of the esophagus and tracheobronchial aspiration" (Berman and Kirsner, 1972a). Most individuals with hiatus hernia respond well to a program with attention to weight reduction, small bland meals, antacids, no tight clothes and elevation of the head of the bed during sleep.

Stomach. Gastric motility may decrease slightly with age, and there is an apparent reduction of hunger contractions (Ivy and Grossman, 1952). Atrophic gastritis is usually asymptomatic, but biopsy slides show an incidence of 3.7% in the 21-30 age group and an incidence of 16.2% in the over 70 (Joske et al., 1955). Concern with this increase relates to a possible predisposition to pernicious anemia plus gastric carcinoma. Achlorhydria may develop, since secretion of HC1 is reduced both in volume and concentration. However, there appears to be a lower incidence of achlorhydria than earlier evaluations suggest (Blackman et al., 1970).

Peptic ulcer appears to be a common problem of the "aging gut." Levrat, et al., (1966) reported that 15% of hospitalized patients for peptic ulcer were 60 years or older. Gastric ulcer is more frequent among older persons than duodenal ulcer. Hemorrhage, perforation, pyloric obstruction, and failure to heal all occur more in the elderly (Cutler, 1958; Levrat et al., 1966). Perhaps the most significant contribution to the development of ulceration are the drugs alluded to earlier: steroids, indomethacin, reserpine, phenylbutazone, and aspirin. All of these are regrettably, too frequently used with and by people over 50 years of age.

Small intestine. Absorptive changes with age in the small intestine are those that significantly interact with nutrition. There is a fall in the absorption of d-xylose (Guth, 1968), vitamins B_1 (Rafsky and Newman, 1948), and folic acid (Hurdle and Williams, 1966). Fat absorption also decreases (Ryder, 1963). There may be poor absorption of calcium as a result of steatorrhea in the older person with postgastrectomy, malabsorption or jejunal diverticulosis. Restrictions in regional blood flow which increase with age probably contribute as well to malabsorptive disorders. The circulatory alterations may develop into chronic ischemia and decreased blood flow to the small bowel (Joske et al., 1958).

Large intestine. The large intestine appears to be of greater concern to the clinicians as well as to the older person. Contrary to earlier thoughts that the colon atrophies, becoming thin and atonic with age, more recent investigations of elderly persons with diverticulosis reveal that there is a thickening of the circular and longitudinal muscle layers of the colon with some weakness of the circular muscle where it intersects with the straight arteries of the sigmoid colon (Morson, 1963).

The high rate of laxatives in use by older persons reflects the widespread existence of constipation. "In one series, people over 70 used laxatives twice as frequently as those in age group from 40-50" (Berman and Kirsner, 1972b). Constipation is observed in 25% of older patients (Portis and King, 1952; Connell et al., 1965). Many factors contribute variously to its development (Hootnick, 1956):

diet: decreased fluid intake, lack of bulk to stimulate peristalsis, poor dentition which decreases food intake.

medication: including sedatives, tranquilizers, anti-hypertensives, ganglionic blocking agents, narcotics and calcium carbonate antacids.

physiology: decreased muscle tone and motor function of bowel.

pathology: muscle spasm of sphincter.
tumor.
prolonged immobilization associated with fractures or paralysis.

PROTEIN, AMINO ACID METABOLISM

Health of elderly women living alone correlated closely with the proportion of protein in the diet (Exton-Smith and Stanton, 1965). An important unanswered question involves the potential of diet therapy and/or rehabilitation of the reduced body mass (muscle and bone) that appears to accompany age. Radioactive potassium studies indicate a continuing loss of tissue beginning at 25 (Forbes and Reina,

1970) estimated to be about 20% of body protein by 65 years of age.

Protein requirement determination. Protein requirements have been arrived at by 2 different methods.

Factorial method

Investigations have determined obligatory N losses by subjects on a protein-free diet. The amount of good quality protein just enough to replace these N losses is then considered the requirement of dietary protein.

Equilibrium study

Subjects are provided with different amounts of good quality protein, and the dietary protein requirement is that minimum which will maintain N equilibrium (about 24g protein for the average 70 kg adult). An additional 30% is added to cover maximum individual requirements (70 mg/kg body weight) up to two standard deviations above the mean (Munro, 1974).

Requirements for the essential amino acids have been determined by feeding a diet of mixed amino acids in place of protein and varying the concentration of one amino acid at a time. The bulk of the data accumulated has used the maintenance of N equilibrium as the criterion. More recently, changes in levels of blood amino acids at different intake concentrations have been used as criteria.

The proportion of dietary essential amino acids is reduced from over 40% in the infant to less than 20% in the adult (Munro, 1972). A majority of food protein contains 40 to 50% essential amino acids and so generally an adult fulfills requirements for total N easily, except if the major source is protein of low biological value such as wheat gluten.

However, with disease, other stress and convalescence (all three frequent in the lives of older persons) the requirements for essential amino acids are closer to those for growth rather than adult maintenance needs.

Energy intake and protein metabolism. The efficient use of amino acids is dependent not only on the quantity and quality of dietary protein, but upon concurrent carbohydrate intake, an action referred to as protein-sparing (from use as a source of energy). Plasma amino acid levels are reduced following a carbohydrate-rich meal. It appears that amino acids are shunted to muscle, a lower supply is available to other tissues and the liver, which consequently produces less protein and urea. Moreover, carbohydrates contribute to the lowering of the non-esterified plasma fatty acids through action of insulin on adipose tissue. However, improved nitrogen sparing has also been demonstrated with glucose-free amino acid infusions in immediate postoperative periods and other catabolic situations (Hoover et al., 1975; Blackburn et al., 1973). There is the suggestion that lowered insulin levels, in response to the glucose-free infusion, stimulate the use of endogenous fat to fulfill energy needs. Of particular note is the fact that isotonic amino acids alone provided protein-sparing considerably beyond that achieved with glucose alone. Addition of hypocaloric glucose or lipid did not create a larger negative N balance. It appears that hypocaloric glucose does not increase mobilization of muscle protein despite the higher insulin concentration. Nitrogen balance was identical with only amino acids, amino acid plus lipid or amino acid plus glucose. It is conceivable that the role of infusions in improving N balance may be a function of both improved protein synthesis and reduced catabolism (Greenberg et al., 1976).

Young et al., in 1972 reported another procedure to test the hypothesis that "not only is there a probable shift in distribution of body protein synthesis with advancing age, but the rate of muscle protein breakdown and synthesis may decline at the same time." (Young et al., 1976 a,b). Urinary excretion of the amino acid 3-methyhistidine, found in actin of all muscles and in myosin of "white" muscle fibers, is compared in young adults and elderly individuals. Unlike most other amino acids of body proteins, it is not recycled for protein synthesis and its urinary concentration can be used as a measure of the "rate and extent of muscle protein breakdown in human subjects" (Young et al., 1973 a,b).

Preliminary results, based on only a few individuals, indicate that daily output of 3-methylhistidine is much lower in the elderly than in young adults, an expected finding in view of decreased muscle mass. With correction for differences in creatinine excretion, the urinary output of 3-methylhistidine is still different for the two age groups. The rate of muscle protein breakdown does, therefore, decrease with advanced age. In the young adult, it represents the daily breakdown of 150 gms of muscle protein; in the elderly, 50 gms (Young et al., 1976).

Prolonged intake of protein-deficient diets have been shown to retard the development and affect the composition of brain. Such malnutrition may result in long term behavioral and learning deficits. Recently, it has been demonstrated that "rapid and specific changes in brain composition normally occur after each meal" (Wurtman and Fernstrom, 1974, p. 193). The neurotransmitter, serotonin, and its amino acid precursor tryptophan, increase in response to particular food intake.

Earlier, Wurtman et al., (1968), reported that concentrations of tryptophan and most amino acids in human plasma demonstrate "characteristic and parallel" fluctuations during each 24 hour period; tryptophan is lowest between 2 to 4 A.M., at 50 to 80% of plateau in the morning. Plasma amino acid rhythms, though not only the result of cyclic ingestion of dietary protein, disappeared in subjects on a total fast, indicating the importance of nutritional intake. For example, insulin in response to dietary carbohydrate, could participate in the elevation or decline of the plasma amino acids by stimulating their movement into muscle and or other intracellular compartment.

It has been shown that groups of amino acids (neutral, acidic, basic) are carried to the brain by specific carrier systems, and that member amino acids compete for transport sites. Rats fasted overnight and presented with protein mixtures containing 18% casein did not exhibit an increase in plasma tryptophan. In order to pursue the mechanism of the result, two diets were then used — one synthetic with carbohydrates, fats and all amino acids (as in an 18% casein diet), and the other minus five of the amino acids that are potential competitors for the same transport system with tryptophan (i.e. tyrosine, phenyhalanine, leucine, isoleucine and valine). Both diets increased plasma tryptophan above fasting level, but there were *large* increases in brain tryptophan and serotonin only when other amino acids were deleted from the diet.

There may be important consequences to the realization that diet can control brain composition and therefore behavior. It is conceivable that the plasma amino acid pattern detected by the serotonin-releasing brain neurons, transduce this information to neural signals resulting in the increased or decreased release of serotonin (Wurtman and Fernstrom, 1974).

In summary, the details for mechanisms and requirements in protein metabolism are not yet sorted out. This should not come as a surprise with the consideration of the large number of factors intimately involved, first in the dietary components: level of protein intake, amino acid composition of protein, energy intake, food processing and preparation, other dietary constituents and second in the characteristics of the person: age, sex, genetic makeup, psyche and pathology (Young et al., 1976).

LIPID METABOLISM

Fats contribute palatibility to foods and act as a seasoning or spread. They are slowly digested, delaying the emptying of the stomach and therefore contribute to feelings of satiety. In the diet they represent the most concentrated source of energy (approximately 4 kcalories per gram). Fats supply essential fatty acids and are the carriers for the fat-soluble vitamins A,D,E, and K.

There are some foods that are almost entirely fat, e.g. butter, margarine, shortening and cooking oils – ('visible fats') – and contribute about 45% of the dietary fats in developed countries. Fats in foods such as cream, cheese, meat, poultry, fish, nuts, and chocolates contain 20 to 70% fat, whole grain cereals 2 to 9% and seeds 4 to 17%, and are the 'invisible' or hidden fats (Robson et al., 1972). Over 98% of lipids in diets are triglycerides (neutral or true fats). About 31% of fatty acids in dietary fats are palmitic and stearic, 40% monounsaturated fatty acid, oleic, and about 12% are polyunsaturated fatty acids – mainly linoleic.

Digestion of fats involves both chemical and physical processes. Ingested fat in the stomach is freed from protein (to which it is frequently bound), by action of proteolytic enzymes. A coarse emulsion is formed in the stomach and from there this bolus moves into the duodenum to be mixed with bile and pancreatic juices.

Absorption of lipids into cells is achieved in two ways. The first metabolic path yields fatty acids and monoglycerides that result from the hydrolysis of the emulsified fat. They are incorporated directly into the membrane of the intestinal cell. In the second method, the fatty acids and monoglycerides combine with bile salts to form a micelle which facilitates absorption. Triglycerides are resynthesized from glycerol, monoglycerides, diglycerides and fatty acids, and carried in the blood attached to proteins. Triglycerides are synthesized primarily in the liver. In some individuals increased synthesis of triglycerides from carbohydrates in the intestinal mucosal cell results in hypertriglyceridemia.

Changes with age: Changes in lipid transport occur both in relation to age and in relation to obesity.

Cholesterol increases gradually with age in males up to 50 years of age and then declines. In females, the increase peaks at about 60 years of age. In the Tecumseh study (Montoye et al., 1966), a cross-sectional investigation, these differences were confirmed. It is conceivable, as with a similar inquiry concerning body weight, that individuals (particularly males) with a higher cholesterol dropped out of the population because of earlier disease and death.

Serum triglycerides appear to behave in a similar fashion. There is a gradual increase in plasma triglycerides with age in males, reaching a peak at 45 to 50, then a decline. In females, the gradual increase (at lower levels than males) with age peaks at age 55 to 60. This pattern (in males and females) was observed in a study in Stockholm (Carlson and Bottiger, 1972) and in Seattle (Goldstein et al., 1973 a,b). The latter investigation showed that "in a composite graph of serum cholesterol, serum triglyceride and body weight plotted against age, the curves are superimposable" (Bierman, 1973).

Bierman (1976) suggests that increased triglyceride synthesis results in hypertriglyceridemia based on the following sequelae:

- obesity triggers insulin antagonism in tissues that metabolize glucose

- consequently, pancreas puts out more insulin
- insulin is in the perfusing liver, increases endogenous triglyceride synthesis

A relationship between body weight and plasma triglycerides levels was also found. Albrink et al., (1962) found that normal males from 30 to 70 years of age who added more than 10 pounds after 25, had higher triglyceride levels than those who did not gain weight. An experimental study of obesity (Sims and co-workers, 1971) used thin male penitentiary volunteers paid to gain weight. The increase in weight and fat tissue was interpreted as a typical pattern for middle-aged men. There was, as in the studies mentioned earlier, an increase in insulin, triglyceride and cholesterol with an increase in weight.

Rates of cholesterol synthesis also increase with obesity. Population data demonstrate that fattest individuals have higher cholesterol levels (Montoye, 1966), true for males, and somewhat less definitive for females. The Framingham study, in which various parameters were measured of the whole population of a town in Massachusetts, followed the subjects over 15 years (Kannel, 1973). In the follow-up data, it was clear there was a direct relationship between the amount of weight gained and the degree of increase in serum cholesterol level. In those individuals who lost weight, there was a concomitant fall in serum cholesterol.

Obesity does change with age (as discussed elsewhere): specifically, there is an increased proportion of adipose tissue at the expense of lean body mass. Although most investigations to date indicate that the peaking of body weight in middle years is followed by a decline, there is always the possibility that the most obese, who are most likely to become ill early, die earlier and are not part of the older population under study. Obesity appears to exert a significant influence in fuel metabolism in relation to cholesterol, triglyceride and glucose metabolism (to be discussed in detail elsewhere).

Obesity is also implicated in the development of age-related diseases such as maturity onset diabetes and atherosclerosis. The resulting insulin antagonism stimulates high insulin levels. Heightened synthesis of triglyceride and cholesterol lead to increased concentration of circulating triglycerides and lipid deposition in arteries. In time, this latter process results in atherosclerosis. With many years of obesity, an exhausted pancreas provides a decreasing level of insulin. Initially, there follows a glucose intolerance, then basal hyperglycemia and ultimately clinical diabetes (Bierman, 1976). As the diabetic state continues, lipoprotein removal from the blood becomes faulty, causing further hyperlipidemia and exacerbation of the atherosclerosis.

It would appear that a number of factors, endogenous (genetic and others) and environmental, interact over the years to bring about changes in lipid (and carbohydrate) metabolism. These changes may support the development of diabetes and atherosclerosis.

$\mathscr{P}atholog{}ies/\mathscr{D}iet$ 5

One of the difficulties in relating diet to disease is the probable long latent period before manifestation of disease, e.g. maturity-onset diabetes and coronary thrombosis are believed to take twenty years or more to develop. Not only is it difficult to evaluate current intake, but it is even more difficult to assess dietary intake over a period of many years.

Another problem arises from the fact that human diseases are not truly reproducible in more common animals. A third limitation relates to the different patterns of growth of the experimental animals we use. Yet another issue grows from the use of human volunteers and the ethical problems related thereto. Human studies also present the problem of supervision of the diet and physical activity. Since budget is always an issue in the attempt to overcome the foregoing weaknesses, studies are frequently tied down to only a relatively few people. And, finally there is the difference between found correlations and the existence of cause and effect. "Association between diet and disease does not prove causality" (Yudkin et al., 1971).

ATHEROSCLEROSIS, CARDIOVASCULAR DISEASE

Atherosclerosis is thought to begin in childhood, but is generally delayed in expression until middle or old age with one or more clinical manifestations: coronary occlusion, stroke, peripheral vascular ischemia, or other relative or total occlusion of large arteries (Hazzard and Knopp, 1976). Ross and Glomset (1974) describe the interaction of many factors in atherogenesis at the cellular and tissue levels including: a traumatized arterial intima, aggregation of platelets at endothelial sites releasing a chemical factor, which in turn stimulates replication of smooth muscle cells; migration of cells through internal elastic lamina which become the central component in atherosclerotic plaque, and the incorporation storage of large amounts of cholesterol esters 'by these cells.

Therefore, in the consideration of the relationship of the diet to atherosclerosis, all the related risk factors plus hereditary predisposition to hyperlipidemia and premature atherosclerosis will have to be considered. Moreover, all the foregoing processes are subject to other physiological variables, including genetic and nutritional aspects.

Data from a number of research perspectives — (epidemiologic, pathologic, clinical and animal research) appear to indicate a major role for nutrition in the etiology of atherosclerosis. Specifically, it is suggested that dietary saturated fat and cholesterol act to influence blood lipids resulting in a massive deposition of fatty substances in blood vessel walls, which with time, result in atherosclerosis. As cholesterol concentration increases, so does the risk.

An International Atherosclerosis Project indicates there are differences in severity of atherosclerosis in the aorta and coronary arteries, and that lesions appear "most frequently in populations which habitually eat foods high in saturated fats and cholesterol" (Stamler, 1975). High blood cholesterol, along with elevated blood pressure and cigarette smoking, remain the most reliable predictors of atherosclerosis. Two major causative factors for hypercholesteremia include dietary saturated fat and cholesterol. Sedentary life styles and rich food intake are generally inevitable precursors to coronary heart disease by way of obesity and a number of biochemical and physiological consequences: hyperlipidemia, hypertension, hyperglycemia and hyperuricemia.

Differences of opinion still exist related to the efficacy of dietary control of serum cholesterol. Although the liver and intestine do synthesize cholesterol at a rate in keeping with hereditary patterns, many studies make a clear statement that there is a definitive correlation between an increase in dietary cholesterol and an increased serum cholesterol level (Goodman and Smith, 1976; Hazzard and Knopp, 1976; Stamler, 1974). The responsiveness of any individual to dietary control of serum cholesterol appears to vary with the hereditary "set point" (Hazzard and Knopp, 1976).

On the other hand, in a study by Alfin-Slater's group at University of California Los Angeles, there were no changes in serum cholesterol after 8 weeks of eating 2 eggs/day, in addition to the normal amount of cholesterol eaten daily. Because the subjects in that inquiry may have represented a biased group,[1] Dr. Slater et al[2] undertook a second (unpublished) study in which they used questionnaire, 3 day diet responses and blood sample data for the information base. The completed results confirmed their earlier conclusion: what the subjects ate did not affect the levels of blood cholesterol.

A most contrary current voice to those who maintain diet is not the primary culprit in the etiology of atherosclerosis (and hypertension, diabetes and tumor growth) is that of Mr. Pritikin of Santa Monica, California. Mr. Pritikin's concepts and empirical studies in nutrition have been receiving increasing attention from both scientific and lay communities. In a personal discussion/interview with Mr. Pritikin (September 3, 1977) we explored some of his current thinking and work with dietary modifications.

The program of the Longevity Research Institute in which Mr. Pritikin holds the position of Director, is

---

[1] Non-smoking, healthy, young individuals with low serum cholesterol; and older men of the Mormon persuasion who are generally healthier than 'average' of the society.

[2] Reported in the Los Angeles Times, June 9, 1977, Part VI, column by Rose Dosti.

educational, practical and experimental. Diversified researchers and physicians staff the small institute. The thematic concern could be described: to investigate the relationships between nutrition/physical exertion and degenerative diseases (heart disease, diabetes, gout, arterial hypertension, atherosclerosis and cerebrovascular disease). Further, the staff has undertaken to implement their program with persons and institutions. Since a number of these diseases are more common among people in their later years, it is useful to become acquainted with the fact and promise of the theory as represented in the activities of the Longevity Center.

It is Pritikin's conviction that the American diet is toxic, that it closes the arteries and increases the incidence of tumor growth. He suggests that in the developed countries, human requirements have been mistakenly based on data from rat nutritional and physiological studies. The characteristics of the rigorous diet recommended by Pritikin are:

Daily Intake

Fat	5 to 10% daily calories (1/8 to 1/4 of American average)
Sugar, honey, etc.	0 grams (American average greater than 100 gm/day)
Salt	1-2 gm. (about 1/10 of American average)
Caffeine	5-10 mg. (American average greater than 400 mg)
Cholesterol	less than 100 mg. (about 1/8 of American average)

(Leonard et al., 1974 p. xiii)

Mr. Pritikin asserts that any information contrary to the 'traditional' academic approach to nutrition is generally ignored, if not disallowed, without judicious, careful examination. According to Pritikin, the so-called corrective nutritional patterns fashionable in America — such as the high protein diets — are based on incomplete, biased information. The emphasis on high protein intake may have serious consequences for an increased incidence of osteoporosis and osteomalacia. A number of studies which he notes (e.g. Linkswiler et al., 1974) indicate the severe negative calcium balance which appears to result from high dietary protein.

One very particular situation relates to atherosclerosis. Early, empirical indications in the literature concerning the etiology and potential prevention/treatment of athero- sclerosis were not readily translated into changed dietary habits. Information on the food rationed war-torn countries in 1944 (with fat intake down to 20% from 40-50% of daily total) was largely set aside; even the 1954 post mortem examinations of Korean veterans killed in battle which indicated that 77% of them had advanced atherosclerosis, did not change the diets of Americans. Mr. Pritikin is among the earliest investigators who stated that atherosclerosis is reversable. In November of 1975, he reported that 12 patients (with advanced atherosclerosis) were able to demon- strate reversal (documented by "before" and "after" angio- grams) with the Pritikin diet — very low or relatively free of fats, cholesterol and refined sugars. Since then, the work of other researchers has confirmed his findings (Barndt et al., 1977; Gresham, 1976). He does not accept the substitution of polyunsaturated fats for the saturated fats as helpful to the individual. According to Mr. Pritikin, the artificial lowering of serum cholesterol which may result is no indication of decreased deposition of lipid substances within the blood vessel walls and may, in fact, enhance the deposition.

At the Longevity Center, they have found that two other chronic diseases more prevalent in the middle and later years are susceptible to dietary and exercise intervention. It is Pritikin's promise that "80% of all diabetics and hyper- tensives within the country would be free of symptoms and off all medication within 90 days of the adoption of the diet and exercise regimen" recommended by his program.

A completed study with the Center's first 650 patients (from January 1976 through April 1977) is being analyzed at this time by a scientific staff of the University at Loma Linda Medical School. Altogether about 1,000 persons have completed 26 day stays at the Institute — most of them with a physical ailment of one kind or another. Five percent of their clients to date have been relatively well individuals who have come to learn the 'diet and exercise regimen' for what they perceive as prevention. The Center is now raising funds to begin their first 'controlled experimental inquiry': a 3 to 5 year study with 1,400 couples of a leisure village, 55 years and older. Members of the institute staff will live 'on the campus' of the village with the couples to carry through on the diet and exercise methodology, while the medical and research staffs of Loma Linda and University of California at Davis will make the random selection and all the objective biochemical, physical and physiological measurements. The scientific community will then have an opportunity to examine the methodology and results on the basis of an apparently reproducible, testable design.

In Finland (Turpeinen, 1968) where coronary heart disease (CHD) mortality is the highest in the world, they have concentrated almost completely on diet control. They are also aware of the multifactorial bases of CHD prevention. In their trials the "lipid hypotheses" was validated:

1. Saturated fatty acids were decreased, polyunsaturates were increased.

2. A fall in plasma cholesterol was maintained at a moderately constant level while on the diet.

3. Adipose tissue contained nearly three times as much polyunsaturated fats. However, when persons discontinued the diets, composition of adipose tissue was almost completely reversed in three years.

4. New "coronary events" were noticeably less in persons adhering to the diet. When they returned to previous "normal" diet, incidence increased.

5. Death from CHD was considerably lower during the diet periods.

6. They found no consistent increase in mortality from malignant neoplasms in patients on the diet.

Dr. Turpeinen's emphasis on the dietary approach does not exclude other promising avenues. He added that Finland also needs to pursue most energetically, a fight against cigarette smoking, lack of exercise, and stress. It is his opinion "that the food industry could play a most important role by producing more low-fat or modified-fat foods —

perfectly feasible from a technical and economic standpoint."

Exactly how dietary low-cholesterol and unsaturated fats lower serum cholesterol is a mechanism awaiting discovery. Blood tryglyceride level is considered a good predictor of atherosclerosis. Macdonald of London (1974) considers that dietary carbohydrate plays an important role in tryglyceride levels – ultimately a portion of high dietary carbohydrates is converted to fat in the blood.

The role of dietary carbohydrates is important since a diet high in carbohydrates raises the fasting serum triglyceride level. More fructose than glucose is converted into serum triglyceride and sucrose contains fructose. The liver can convert fructose to glucose, but possibly only when large quantities of glucose are consumed (Macdonald, 1975).

Macdonald emphasizes that the lipid response to dietary carbohydrate involves other variables as well:

1. *Type of fat consumed with the carbohydrate.* If the fat intake is polyunsaturated, the physiological rise in serum triglycerides after a meal containing fat is reduced by adding carbohydrate (especially glucose) to the meal.

2. *Sex differences.* Atherosclerosis occurs infrequently in premenopausal women compared to men in the same age group. Triglyceride elevation from sucrose or fructose does not occur in young women as it does in young men. Oral contraceptives plus dietary sucrose raise the triglyceride level higher than do either alone.

3. *Frequency.* The frequency of consumption of large quantities of sucrose and the N source accompanying sucrose alter the triglyceride level.

Carbohydrate sensitivity is measurable with serum triglyceride levels after a 12-14 hour fast. If positive, reduction of dietary carbohydrate is indicated. Along with this reduction, more polyunsaturated fats will also help to offset the effect of dietary carbohydrates. As mentioned elsewhere, weight reduction also helps to eliminate "carbohydrate sensitivity." In his recommendations, Macdonald advises a reduced carbohydrate and an increased polyunsaturate fat intake, in addition to a low-cholesterol diet.

In relation to atherosclerosis and to coronary heart disease, many other studies cited in Hazzard and Knopp (1976), Goodman and Smith (1976) and in *Atherosclerosis* by Medcom (1974), address themselves to common concepts: a diet low in cholesterol and saturated fat, moderate body weight and moderate exercise. There is agreement: (1) that it is possible to screen for and identify risk factors related to premature atherosclerosis and potential CHD, (2) that it is possible to gather quantitative data from epidemiological studies, (3) that with age, hyperlipidemia is less of a major risk factor, (4) that the "typical" Western nutritional intake is characterized by excess calories and animal fat and that diet is a critical factor in the etiology and prevention of atherosclerosis and coronary heart disease, and (5) that there is also widespread agreement that these age-related diseases are multifactorial in origin, and for optimum control these variables need to be addressed in the early years.

The complexity of susceptibility to atherosclerosis and CHD is highlighted in stark relief in the study of the Masai tribesmen of Eastern Africa (Mann and Spoerry, 1974). They are unusually resistant to heart disease although their diet is essentially milk and meat, both very high in cholesterol and saturated fats. Ordinarily the Masai, tall and lean, have very low blood cholesterol levels, 135 mg/100 ml of blood. However, the Masai also walk up to 35 miles a day and do not contend with the degree and kind of stress typical of Western contemporary society.

There are suggestions in the literature of the importance of other dietary factors in the etiology of cardiovascular disease, namely, trace elements. Since 1957, data suggest that the harder the drinking water, the lower the mortality from cardiovascular disease. The protective effect of hard water appears to be due mainly to Ca^{++} and Mg^{++} content (Somogyi, 1975). This area of inquiry has recently emerged and the level of sophistication is low. At this point, the few accounts are descriptive and tentatively speculative.

CANCER, DIET AND THE ALIMENTARY TRACT

Epidemiologists continue to pursue the relationships which appear to exist between dietary factors and cancer of the alimentary tract (NUTRITION REVIEWS, 1973).

Most researchers agree it is reasonable to theorize an important role for fiber. Some of the thinking is focused on the delay in fecal elimination, which has developed due to the decrease in fiber consumption in the past 25 years (Burkitt et al., 1972). The argument continues that if a cancer agent (virus or chemical) gains access to the intestine, there is more time for damage to take place in the gut on a low fiber diet than on a high fiber diet (Scala, 1974).

Fiber also contributes to the increase of water, sterols, bile acids, and fats, all of which could have a combined solvent-like effect to eliminate any toxic substances (Burkitt, 1971).

Nutrition and diet are thought to influence carcinogens in either of two ways: food or drink which may be the carriers of carcinogens; a diet whose composition stimulates the kind of enzymatic activity and other changes which may yield tumors (Clayson, 1975). "In animals, caloric restriction, type and amount of dietary fat, deficiencies of certain vitamins and minerals and dietary protein and amino acids all influence induction or growth of tumors" (DAIRY COUNCIL DIGEST, Sept./Oct. 1975). Epidemiological studies with human populations have emphasized the roles of high fat intake or lack of fiber in breast and colon cancer (Lea, 1966; Wynder et al., 1969).

A higher incidence of fatal carcinomas was reported in a group of persons with a diet containing four times as much polyunsaturated fatty acids (PUFA) and half as much cholesterol as a conventionally fed group (Pearce and Dayton, 1971). Mechanisms for action in relation to carcinogenesis have been discussed. Rose et al., (1974), suggest that high PUFA could stimulate increased bile salt formation, providing more substrate for the carcinogen-forming bacteria. An inhibition of the antigen-induced lymphocyte response by PUFA is reported by Mertin (1973). This inhibition interferes with "immune surveillance capacity" and aberrant cells which normally would be removed from the circulation may now remain.

The literature relating vitamin deficiencies to carcinogenesis is equivocal, some deficiencies appear to enhance, others to suppress (DAIRY COUNCIL DIGEST, Sept./Oct.

1975). Some minerals have likewise been implicated in tumor development and increased mortality from cancer (Cameron and Pauling, 1973), and deficiencies of others have been suggested as related to increased incidence (Shils, 1973).

There is widespread support for the notion that diverticular disease, called endemic in the last half of life by Painter and Burkitt (1971), and possibly colorectal cancer may be prevented by avoidance of fiber low foods, white flour, sugar and high-fat containing foods.

It is relatively clear that the older individual remains more susceptible to neoplasia of the digestive tract than the younger persons. What is not clear, is whether some of the functional and moderate anatomical changes in the gastro-intestinal tract with age are normal concomitants of age or the imposition of disease. Additional data about the morphological and functional changes of gastrointestinal tract with age would appear to be a major priority.

This "tube" within the body has the responsibility all through the lifespan for supplying digested nutrients. These must be absorbed via a large mucosal surface lining the lumen, and integrated into the multiple metabolic paths unique to each individual. What is hopeful is an apparently majority suggestion that intervention in the form of changing nutritional habits may restore or maintain the digestive system in good function in the last half of life.

CANCER AND NUTRITIONAL DEFICIENCY

The incidence of most cancers increase with age; about one half of all cancer deaths take place in the over 65 (Smith and Bierman, 1973). One of the environmental factors that has been raised as a potential contributor to increased vulnerability to cancer is nutrition. A brief look at whatever data are in the literature identifies another direction for further investigation. There are researchers who maintain that cancer is a nutritional deficiency disease. The claim continues . . . if the body is healthy and all cells functioning well, cancerous cells will not be activated. In addition, some workers in the field state that prevention of cancer is possible with an optimal diet. "Evidence suggests that nutrition affects the incidence of a large portion of human cancers, perhaps relating to as much as 50% of all cancers in woman and one third of all cancers in men." So spoke Ernst L. Wynder in his opening remarks at the Symposium on Nutrition in Causation of Cancer, sponsored by the National Cancer Institute and the American Cancer Society in Florida, May 1975 (Long, 1976, Wynder et al., 1961).

For example, in states of wound repair, inflammation, and cancer, a patient appears to be deficient in ascorbic acid; total body requirements have become abnormally high (Cameron and Pauling, 1973). It is their theoretical position that vitamin C may be effective in the inhibition of the enzyme, hyaluronidase, (implicated in growth of cancerous tissue) secreted by viruses, bacteria and cancerous cells.

In the experimental animal, Sporn and colleagues (1976) found that vitamin A deficiency enhanced susceptibility to chemical carcinogens introduced into the respiratory system, the bladder and the colon. These same investigators, in a study of more than 8,000 men in Norway, found there was a correlation between a realtively low vitamin A intake and a high incidence of lung cancer (Long, 1976). Vitale (1975) concluded that cancer "may be preventable to a large degree by manipulation of the diet, environment, or microbial flora." It has been noted that an infectious agent may take hold when the host and the agent compete for available iron, as well as for other nutrients (Lepshitz et al., 1971).

Healthy body cells derive energy from foods most efficiently by way of oxidative (oxygen-dependent) respiration. Cancer cells use anaerobic (fermentation) metabolism, typical of a system deprived of oxygen as in anemia and hypothyroidism. The series of cell reactions (Krebs cycle) unique to aerobic respiration, require adequate vitamins and minerals to sucessfully continue the oxidative activities for energy and metabolite production. The connection with good nutritional status is clearcut.

Examination of cells in nutritionally deficient cell suspensions, small animal tissue and human sera and biopsies, provide evidence of the deterioration of form (and inevitably, function) that appears to follow continued inadequate nutrient intake. Cell organelles are affected in a variety of ways which have been correlated with nutritional insufficiency: an increase in aberrant mitochondria but a decrease in their total number; disrupted lysosomal, mitochondrial and plasma membranes; distorted nuclei and increased vacuoles. Malnutrition also is correlated with a decreased efficiency of the immune system. The reduced energy and nutrients result in diminished protein synthesis which leads to low antibody (a protein) production, and fewer, slower acting leucocytes (Hayflick, 1975; Scrimshaw, 1964; Vitale, 1975).

These kinds of data are primarily suggestive and experimental in nature, not always the results of controlled, reproducible regimens. Nevertheless, research in this area is essential and could conceivably answer some important questions. Data could lead to much needed preventive and therapeutic approaches related to malignancy. The question remains essentially unanswered: does a deficient diet leave the individual more vulnerable to cancerous invasion?

DIVERTICULOSIS/DIVERTICULITIS

In 1967, Manousos and associates determined that 40% of people over 70 in the Oxford area had diverticulosis. Estimates for diverticula range from 20% of persons over 40 to 40% in persons over 70, or 30-40% of population over 60 in Great Britain (Almy, 1977; Strode, 1968). There is no adequate survey of the prevalence of diverticulosis in the United States, but it is probable that disability from this cause affects between 5 and 10% of those over 60 years (Almy, 1977). In general, diverticula of the colon is of small note as long as there are no particular symptoms. But diverticular disease has become a major deficiency disease of western civilization (Painter and Burkitt, 1971). Some clinicians identify the excessive thickening of the colonic muscle, with consequent bowel segments and increased intraluminal pressure, as the "underlying pathogenic mechanism" (Berman and Kirsner, 1972 b).

Diverticulitis (inflammation, infection accompanying diverticulosis) usually results from the perforation of a single diverticulum and is said to be increasing at a rate as high at 16% (Scala, 1974). Straining is one of the characteristics of diverticular persons, resulting in excessive pressure in the venous system of the large intestine and legs. Hemorrhoids and varicose veins follow close, yet both of these are susceptible to an increase in dietary fiber (Painter, et al., 1972).

Increasingly, researchers and clinicians support the hypothesis that diverticulosis may be caused by a deficiency of vegetable fiber in the diet. Nutrition is, therefore, a major consideration in the prevention and treatment of this disease (Painter and Burkitt, 1971; Hodkinson, 1972). Further, this roughage deficiency is seen as due primarily to an overconsumption of refined carbohydrates. The disease in western countries appears to increase in direct proportion to the increased intake of refined carbohydrates. Large, more watery stools that result from high residue diet produce less pressure and a larger colon diameter, both factors in a lower incidence of diverticula. 80% of older persons treated with bran experienced successful relief of symptoms (Painter and Burkitt, 1971).

There are numerous references in the literature to 'functional bowel disease' (Freeman, 1965; Sklar, 1970) as probably the most common among older persons. Symptomology includes constipation, diarrhea, distension, abdominal pain and excessive mucous in bowel movements. More often than not, a significant role is played by emotional problems which plague many older persons: loneliness, depression, boredom, a diminished sense of self, and fear of disease. Fatigue, dietary excesses, excessive use of laxatives and enemas add to the level of stress already created. These are all compounded by the lowered income and the drop in the standard of living that marks the later years of so many in America today.

DIABETES

Research has demonstrated that simple lack of insulin is far from being the entire issue in diabetes. Increasingly, biochemical investigations have yielded additional evidence. However, the primary underlying defect in diabetes is not known at this time. Diabetes may be classified into three major types:

1. *Pancreatic* — occurs with destruction of islet cell tissue

by inflammation, infiltrative lesions or surgical removal.

2. *Endocrine* — produced by an excess of a hormone or hormones that antagonize or oppose the action of insulin. This type is usually very mild.

3. *Idiopathic* — (of unknown origin) the most common clinical type, occurs in two forms: Juvenile or growth-onset diabetes, in patients less than 40 years of age, often is rapid in onset and produces ketosis.

Some authorities believe that the pattern of inheritance in diabetes is of a Mendelian recessive type, but with incomplete penetration of the trait. Studies of twins suggest the involvement of other factors in the development of diabetes, since even identical twins are not similarly affected — only about one half are demonstrably diabetic (Davies, 1975). Obesity and age are considered etiological factors in maturity onset diabetes (idiopathic) which is more common in women than in men. Recent evidence suggests the incidence is increasing in men, and the sex ratio may be changing (Pyke, 1968). Moreover, iatrogenic factors have been increasingly associated with the deterioration of glucose tolerance and potential diabetes: exogenous steroids, contraceptive steroids, and thiazide diuretics (Davies, 1975).

The maturity-onset or adult type usually occurs in patients more than forty years old, is frequently slow in onset, relatively resistant to ketosis, and usually responds to oral hypoglycemic agents and/or dietary control. This suggests that islet cells may retain the capacity to produce insulin, but at inadequate levels.

The work of Andres and Tobin (1975) is primarily concerned with the differentiation of a normal age change from a diseased state — in relation to the effect of age on carbohydrate metabolism. By 1978, the study of diabetes at the Gerontology Research Center in Baltimore will have been in progress for 13 years (begun in 1965). The persons under study are a group of 600 male volunteers who live in the greater Washington, D.C. area, 17-103 years or more of age, healthy, highly educated and in the upper middle class. They agreed to return for testing every 18 months for the rest of their lives, for 2½ days each visit, and live at the Baltimore City Hospitals. One of five tests in the diabetes sphere is conducted at each visit: oral glucose tolerance, cortisone tolerance, intravenous tolbutamide tolerance and the glucose clamp's study.

There would appear to be consensus among researchers and clinicians (Andres and Tobin, in press) concerning the following:

1. There is a deterioration of 'tolerance' — the decreased capacity to handle administered glucose efficiently is progressive throughout the adult lifespan.
2. A variety of diagnostic tests for diabetes all show this age effect.
3. The deterioration of performance is so large that approximately half of older subjects lie above an arbitrary mean + 2 standard deviations.

Major questions of considerable theoretical and clinical importance exist, and are still surrounded by marked differences of opinion:

1. Should age adjustments of normality be made or should all subjects be judged by standards derived from young adults?
2. Is the mechanism of deterioration in performance (with age) identical with, similar to or entirely different from the mechanism underlying the disease, diabetes mellitus?
3. In a quantitative sense, just how common is the deterioration of performance? (Some reports indicate only a slight change with age, others report that 100% of older subjects are abnormal).
4. The overriding basic question: Is the change with age physiologic, adaptive (i.e. normal) or pathologic (the emergence of a pathological harmful disease)?

There are many variables that may be responsible for the diverse estimates of 'abnormality.'

1. In the performance of diagnostic tests.
2. In the techniques used to select young and old subjects.
3. Technical variables: dose of glucose, blood sampling times, time of day of administration, physical activity during test, use of venous or capillary blood measure-

ment of glucose concentration in whole blood, plasma or serum, and the chemical methods for glucose analysis.

A decision as to "normality" or "abnormality" of various percentiles is at this time arbitrary. The derivation and evaluation of a nomogram is achieved by 'deriving an individual's performance in comparison to his own age cohort and expressed in terms of percentile rank.' Two approaches may be used. One is actuarial and involves long-term follow up of large numbers of individuals over the entire adult life span. The second is experimental with the goal of identification of the mechanism of deterioration. The two questions related to mechanism that help to direct the inquiry are:

1. Is the pancreatic beta cell response to hyperglycemia decreased with advancing age *or* is age secondary to an adequate insulin response?

2. Is sensitivity of tissues to insulin reduced with age *or* is age change secondary to administered sensitivity of body tissues to insulin secreted?

A recently developed technique 'glucose clamp,' to maintain steady state, (Andres et al., 1970) attempts to avoid the problem of uncontrolled concentration of insulin response that has been noted in studies. Blood glucose is monitored continuously by the researcher with rapid analysis of arterial glucose concentration, and controlled by an appropriate feedback servo-control of a continuous, but variable intravenous glucose infusion rate. A steady state hyperglycemia is maintained at four levels 140, 180, 220 and 300 mg/100 ml for 2 hours. This technique results in a biphasic serum insulin response, a rapid peak followed by a fall and a secondary slow rise. Older subjects at the three lower glucose plateaus show miniature insulin curves as compared to the younger. In this technique, the pancrease is perfused slowly with arterial blood, and since the hyperglycemic stimulus to insulin release is identical in all subjects, Andres and Tobin conclude that the results point to the fact that beta cell sensitivity to glucose decreases with age.

It is most important to note that there are hormonal as well as non-hormonal controls of the glucose economy of the body and that the complexities of interaction of all these factors have only been minimally investigated. For example "gastrointestinal stimulating hormones" have been shown to be most important. This is suggested by the greater insulin release from oral administration of glucose as compared to intravenous glucose. Possible age differences and quantitative aspects of this response are unknown (Andres and Tobin 1975).

There have been a number of different techniques to determine an assessment of 'insulin sensitivity' or effectiveness of insulin at its target organ. They have produced discrepant results. The advent of the immunoassay has also provided a remarkable stimulus to research on insulin response. Tobin et al., (1972) use an alternative approach by adapting the 'glucose clamp' technique. In that way they are able to determine sensitivity by measuring the rate of glucose infused under steady state conditions. They found no differences with age.

Proinsulin, a single chain molecule also synthesized in the beta cell, is cleaved intracellularly to form the double chain insulin (Steiner et al., 1972). Proinsulin is also released intact, but its biological potency is only a small fraction of that of insulin. Measurement of serum insulin levels, therefore, may be deceptive. Only one study (Duckworth and Kitabachi, 1972) is reportable:

1. There are no differences in proinsulin levels under basal conditions in humans. After an oral glucose challenge, proinsulin levels rose earlier and higher in 40-60 year old subjects than in 21-35 year olds.

2. By 3 hours after oral glucose, 9% of total immunoreactive insulin (IRI) was proinsulin in younger subjects but 16% in older persons.

Further studies related to proinsulin/insulin ratio are necessary to avoid misinterpretation of the sensitivity of tissues to insulin.

Recent availability of a highly specific immunoassay for glucagon have enabled some investigations of its role in diabetes, but very little related to age and glucagon physiology. The alpha cell hormone of the pancreas, glucagon, may play an important role in pathophysiology of diabetes mellitus (Unger, 1971). Additional aspects of carbohydrate and lipid metabolism in middle aged, physically well trained men (Bjorntorp et al., 1972) has shed some general light. Physical training does appear to elevate maximal oxygen uptake, to lower fasting plasma lipids, and to enhance assimilation of oral glucose, which stimulates much lower insulin than in controls. It was their suggestion that changes in muscle capacity to metabolize glucose may be involved.

An interesting reflection of the Timeline from discovery of new information to its total application is marked in the insulin — carbohydrate diet relationship. The current recommendations of the American Diabetic Association (through its Committee on Food and Nutrition) state that dietary carbohydrate restriction is not necessary for the majority of diabetics (Bierman et al., 1971).

This was known and concluded shortly after insulin came into use (about 50 years ago). Insulin enabled the glucose to be adequately cleared from the blood with little excess spilled into the urine. It would appear that a high carbohydrate diet is even 'desirable' since it may be the most efficient mechanism to lower the dietary cholesterol and saturated fats. In a number of studies, diabetics with a high carbohydrate diet demonstrated an improvement in glucose tolerance (Weinsier et al., 1974). Both cholesterol and saturated fats have been implicated in hyperlipidemia and atherosclerosis, and diabetics are vulnerable to both. The diet is a variable that can be controlled — more attention appears warranted.

CONCLUSIONS/(DIABETES)

1. There is no clear consensus concerning age differences in beta cell sensitivity. In most tests, results vary. But with glucose clamp technique, beta cell sensitivity to hyper-glycemia is decreased in old subjects.

2. Sensitivity of body tissues to endogenously released insulin and exogenous administration is not decreased in old subjects, but a pattern of decreasing sensitivity to insulin in the second hour of study is unique to older persons.

3. Aging is associated with significant decreases in performance in various diagnostic tests for diabetes. Significance
of these age differences remains in dispute.

NUTRITIONAL ANEMIAS

Iron deficiency. Iron deficiency anemia is fairly widespread in the elderly (as indicated by the Hanes Survey).[3]
Dietary iron deficiency and consequent nutritional anemia
are most frequently due to a generally inadequate diet and/or
malabsorption, the latter probably a function of achlorhydria
(Bender, 1971b). However, in a relatively high proportion of
older persons, a slow gastrointestinal bleeding may be
involved, often undetected. This occult intestinal bleeding
(frequently tied to excessive salicylate ingestion or cancer)
has been found to be a major factor in iron deficiency anemia
(MacLennan et al., 1973).

Untreated anemia does result in tissue changes which
can be observed most typically in the fingernails which
become brittle, thin, often peeling and broken. Large areas of
the skin may also become dry and inelastic, the hair thin and
likely to break. Atrophy of the tongue may occur. Unabated
iron deficiency anemia may also result in atrophy and
friability of the esophageal mucosa. Additional obvious
symptoms are shortness of breath, ankle swelling, lack of
appetite, weakness and an overall reduction in the body's
physiological activities. Many of these changes may be due to
impaired nutrition of the tissues as a result of the depletion
of iron containing enzymes necessary for biological oxidation.

The older person who frequently develops anemia is
that person who lives alone, on a reduced income and has lost
interest in cooking and nutritional requirements, and
attempts to live on 'tea and toast' (Clifford, 1971).
Treatment usually makes use of oral iron in medicinal forms

[3] U.S. Department of Health Education and Welfare. Preliminary Findings
of the First Health and Nutrition Examination Survey. United States,
1971-1972; Dietary Intake and Biochemical Findings. DHEW Publication No. (HRA) 74-1219-1.

that have the greatest amount of iron in the reduced state e.g. ferrous sulfate that state which is most readily absorbed. However, more satisfactory is a combination of dietary changes and medicinal therapy (Clifford, 1971; Mayer, 1975a).

An increase in the diet of iron-containing foods e.g. liver, kidney, most meats, nuts, eggs, green leafy vegetables, and enriched or whole grain bread and cereals would increase the iron concentration in the diet. This kind of dietary intake is important to establish, even if iron supplementation is used initially and completed, for the iron in the ingested food will remain available on a long term basis.

Pernicious anemia. Generally unique to later life, is the disease, pernicious anemia. This disturbance may be experienced for the first time in the 10th decade and is responsive to treatment (Agate, 1971). Pernicious anemia differs from iron deficiency anemia; there is a reduction in white cells and platelets as well as the erythrocytic alterations of other anemias. It differs also in its etiology since the basic cause is a vitamin B_{12} deficiency (or malabsorption of dietary B_{12}), it develops later in life, and is probably of genetic origin.

There are some researchers who do suggest that pernicious anemia may be an autoimmune disease. Vitamin B_{12} deficiency not only alters the blood pressure but is correlated with diverse lesions (Clifford, 1971). The multiple metabolic roles of vitamin B_{12} in nucleic acid and lipid synthesis, and in substrate provision to the Kreb's cycle, may account for the widespread symptomology of pernicious anemia. Diagnosis is usually established by metabolic abnormalities, identification of histamine fast achlorhydria and a response to vitamin B_{12} therapy. Lifelong lower dosage maintenance therapy of vitamin B_{12} is generally required and recommended.

Response to treatment by older persons in both iron deficiency and pernicious anemias is excellent and failure to achieve control generally indicates other co-existing factors such as 'occult malignant disorder, undetected intestinal bleeding, chronic infection or poor nutritional status.' These may all impair the body capacity to respond to treatment (Clifford, 1971). Perhaps a particularly important feature of the 'chronic anemias' of the later years, is the essentially unnoticed onset of measurable symptoms and consequent physiological alterations.

Folic acid deficiency anemia (megaloblastic or macrocytic anemia). Folic acid deficiency is the third major cause of nutritional anemia, and may be more widespread than earlier thought. As indicated in the earlier vitamin discussion, folic acid is essential for appropriate DNA synthesis and folate deficiency is often difficult to distinguish from vitamin B_{12} deficiency. There are no large body stores of folic acid (as there is with vitamin B_{12}), so that with inadequate nutrition (particular lack of dark green leafy vegetables and/or beans), folic acid deficiency anemia may develop within 3 to 4 months (Clifford, 1971). Vitamin B_{12} therapy may not have to continue indefinitely and can be stopped when an adequate diet has been achieved and maintained.

OSTEOPOROSIS

Osteoporosis is an entity, a condition resulting from a number of processes that lead to the diminution of bone in the skeleton. It was recognized during the 19th century by German anatomists who distinguished it from osteomalacia (Exton-Smith, 1973). Albright and colleagues (1941) defined it as "too little bone, but what bone there is, is normal."

Osteoporosis probably occurs in one-third of women over the age of 60, and is observable in men and women of younger ages. There are researchers who estimate that 50% of post-menopausal women in the United States have this disease (Smith and Rizek, 1966). Other estimates suggest that at least 10% of persons, (male and female) 55 and older suffer from osteoporosis, advanced enough to cause fractures (Lutwak, 1964). The incidence of "senile" osteoporosis is approximately four times greater in women than in men (Albanese et al., 1975). Others suggest that osteoporosis may be a natural consequence of aging (Newton-John and Morgan, 1968). Age of onset appears to be decreasing. Evidence is, that in general, it is not a dysfunction which develops suddenly in middle or old age, but probably begins gradually at approximately 25 years of age (Rose, 1965).

The definition of the disease is complex. A nonsymptomatic, so-called 'normal' person may have bone loss comparable to a patient with diagnosed osteoporosis, but has not sustained a fracture because no stress has occurred (Jowsey, 1976).

If blood calcium supply is deficient, then bone is resorbed to provide sufficient calcium to maintain serum concentration within the normal range. The parathyroid gland is the site of major control and feedback mechanism essential to sense changes in ionized blood calcium, and to modify the rate of secretion of the hormone. One of the effects of the hormone is to bring about osteoclastic bone resorption which releases calcium and phosphate into the serum, increasing serum Ca++ levels. There are a number of factors to consider in the illumination and treatment of the disease:

1. The amount of bone available at maturity is variable. Cross sectional data suggests that the amount of bone in adult life and old age is determined by skeletal development at maturity. Activity, disease nutrition, endocrine and racial (hereditary) factors need to be evaluated.

2. Females have poorer skeletal development. In general, females have a lower bone mass and this may be an important consideration in the higher incidence of osteoporosis among women.

3. Post-menopausal bone loss is measurable. There appears to be a rapid loss during the first 10 years after the menopause in some women (Gryfe et al., 1971).

4. Pathological conditions.
   a. In some patients, an acute disease process accelerates osteoporosis (Dent and Watson, 1966). Negative Ca++ balance has been demonstrated easily during these 'attacks.'
   b. Immobilization due to fracture, joint disease, splinting and hemiplegia (Hodkinson and Brain, 1967) is accompanied by osteoporosis. The extent to which this process can be reversed is in question: Rose (1970) believes bone remineralization does not occur, Whedon (1970) has shown that it does.
   c. Hyperadrenocorticism. Osteoporosis is fairly common

in persons with Cushing's disease. It also develops in persons treated for years with corticosteroids for rheumatoid arthritis, asthma and skin diseases.
  d. Rheumatoid arthritis. There is a fairly common association of this disease with osteoporosis unrelated to the treatment modality.
  e. Periodontal disease. More recently, interest has developed in periodontal disease, which leads to the loss of teeth in approximately 35 million people in this country, most of whom are older persons (National Center for Health Statistics, Series 11, 1970). Periodontitis may be an early or concomitant expression of osteoporosis. Lutwak et al., (1971) tested the hypothesis that human periodontal disease represents a type of nutritional osteoporosis in a pilot study with 90 unselected 'patients.' Preliminary evidence suggests there is an average increase of 12% in bone density over a 12 month evaluation period in that group receiving a dietary supplement of 1.0 g. of calcium per day. It is theorized that the strength of supporting bone is of major importance in the development of periodontitis.

5. Nutritional factors. Lutwak suggests that "chronic dietary deficiency of calcium and chronic dietary excess of phosphorous results in bone demineralization" (Lutwak, 1976, P. 80 and P. 145).

  a. Calcium deficiency. While many reports maintain there is no calcium deficiency involved, other studies disagree. Lutwak (1976) is of the opinion that increased dietary calcium can be used to prevent resorption of bone.
  b. Vitamin D deficiency. According to Bullamore et al., (1970) a fall in calcium absorption occurs after 70 — which may in part be due to vitamin D deficiency. Correction of the deficiency promotes calcium absorption.
  c. Vitamin C deficiency. Ascorbic acid is necessary for collagen synthesis. Low ascorbic acid levels in the leucocytes are commonly present in old people, but the extent of involvement is not yet known.

d. Protein deficiency. In a nutrition survey in Great Britain (1972) bone mass of the second metacarpal was unrelated to the dietary protein intake in old age. Protein deficiency appears to be "a rare cause of osteoporosis" (Jowsey, 1976).
e. 'Acid-ash' diet. Bone densities of vegetarians were found to be significantly greater than those of individuals whose diet was high in 'acid-ash' (meat eaters) or than the omnivores whose bone density decreased more with age.
f. Fluoride. Evidence from epidemiological studies concerning osteoporosis and fluoride is conflicting. Experimentally, it has been demonstrated that increased dietary fluoride causes greater crystallinity of the bone material. Jowsey (1976) presents a combined treatment of fluoride and calcium in those who have not been treated prophylactically.
g. Calcium/phosphorous ratio. In human bone, the ratio of calcium to phosphorous is 2:1, but phosphorous is higher in soft tissues. Generally, therefore, in approximating the most appropriate dietary ratio, the phosphorous requirement is considered equal to or greater than the allowance for calcium at all age levels except for the young. There appears to be a decreased efficiency in calcium absorption with age, which is also affected by the ratio of dietary calcium to phosphorous. Since milk consumption has decreased, while meat intake remains relatively high or increased, the calcium/phosphorous ratio approaches 1:4 today (Lutwak, 1976). This in contrast to the 1:1 or 2:1 ratios of the average, more balanced diet.

Calcium depletion in animals is enhanced by high levels of dietary phosphorous (Hegsted, 1973) and vice versa. It is not yet clear that this kind of influence can be demonstrated in human nutrition.

Many dietary surveys indicate an average adult consumption of 400 mg of calcium each day — with a range of absorption between 10 and 50%. Since losses each day approximate 270 mg, there could easily be a negative calcium balance of 90 mg. With approximately 1500 grams of calcium in the skeleton at 20 years of age, and a negative calcium balance of 980 grams of calcium by age 50, approximately one-third of the skeletal calcium may remain (Lutwak, 1976). Jowsey (1976) maintains that adequate dietary calcium is an initial important step in the prevention of osteoporosis and that fluoride and calcium may constitute the most effective treatment once the disease is present.

At present, a number of the researchers appear to minimize the role for estrogen in therapeutic regimens. (Lutwak, 1974, 1976; Jowsey, 1976; Exton-Smith, 1973). In some studies, estrogens administered for long periods do not have a significant effect on the total retention of calcium by the skeleton (Lutwak, 1966; Riggs et al., 1972).

Age related bone loss, as seen in osteoporosis and periodontal disease, appears in sum to be a function, not of any single pathological or aging process, but rather a result of a number of interacting changes with time (Garn, 1975). Overlaid on a genetic base, the effects of neuronal, hormonal, gastrointestinal, renal and nutritional activities may be subject to intervention at preventive levels in the early years and rehabilitative levels later.

Behavioral Changes 6

TASTE CAPACITY/FOOD INTAKE

As the psychological and physiological point of entry of the digestive system, taste capacity changes with age may be significant. Taste sensitivity frequently determines the kinds of food in the daily diet and will in the long run affect the overall nutritional status of older persons.

In 1940, Richter and Campbell found that the taste threshold for sucrose among persons 52-85 years old was three times higher than that of the 15-19 age group. A sharp decline after the late 50's in sensitivity for all four basic qualities: sweet, sour, salty, or bitter (Cooper et al., 1959; Kaplan, 1965) was not accompanied by a deterioration in taste sensitivity unless combined with a subject's smoking habits. There was no evidence of general decline in taste sensitivity among 50 persons (60-90 years); a few old people showed marked impairment which the researchers considered pathological (Byrd and Gertman, 1959). More recently, Glanville et al., (1964), concluded that there is a taste threshold increase with age, but found males deteriorated more quickly than females in this respect. Hughes (1969) also found progressive elevation in taste threshold for each decade forward from 60.

Several authors report a decrease in the number of taste nerve endings with age. Arey et al., (1935) compared the taste buds per papilla of children and persons from 74-85: there was a reduction from 248 taste buds per papilla to 83 per papilla; also noted was the atrophy of one-half of the total buds, a reduction of 80% compared with the younger group. These data, though moderately conflicting, do suggest a decline in taste and smell receptors with time, more significant after 60 than before. It appears, then, that heightened flavoring with a conscious avoidance of the addition of empty calories would be a useful approach to adequate nutrition in the last half of life. Bender (1971), from his own investigation of 200 persons aged 10-90+, suggests that the decreased taste sensation of the elderly may have to be taken into account in the formulation of any nutritional product for older persons.

GENERAL ATTITUDES, BELIEFS, PRACTICES

"It's not age that interferes with nutrition of the elderly," so said Dr. Sebrell in 1966. More likely than age or the physiological changes as primary variables, he points to a lifetime of bad habits, mistakes, accidents and diseases. Changing physiology is, nevertheless, a reality.

Early experience. A group of elderly patients provided interesting confirmation of the role of early experience in building of attitudes and behavior about food. Offered a choice of reconstituted frozen orange juice, freshly squeezed orange juice or whole oranges, preference was for the whole orange, then fresh juice, and last for the reconstituted (Sebrell, 1966). Frozen orange juice, a comparatively recent innovation, was obviously not a part of their early experience.

Physiology. A number of older persons tend to avoid meat, milk, many fruits and vegetables (bulk and micronutrients) because of poor teeth, no teeth or ill-fitting prostheses. This in turn may contribute to a sluggish bowel and may account for a considerable percentage of the malnutrition and constipation that plague older persons. There is also the suggestion that some of these diet deficiencies may play a role in the etiology of malignancy.

Enjoyment of food may be diminished with the decrement in the senses of smell and taste, thus eliminating in part the psychic stimulus which initiates the flow of saliva and gastric digestive juices.

Other environmental factors. Other environmental factors in the world of older persons modulate attitudes and practices in relation to food. Low incomes tend to make for increased dietary carbohydrates, (primarily refined sugars) a poor substitute for the essential proteins, fresh fruits and vegetables. Limited food budgets would serve better if smaller portions were packaged and reasonably priced. Living alone exacerbates the constraints of a low budget. Well-balanced meals are rarely prepared on a regular sustaining basis for one person. Any existing pathology further modifies interest in food, affects the way in which the body is able to metabolize food and interferes with efforts to plan and carry out a program for adequate nutrition.

The patterns and attitudes. A study of food behavior of an older population in a South Minneapolis housing development included a random sample of 144 persons on a low income with an average age of 74.5 years (Noble, 1969). Food preferences were found to be set during a lifetime of eating habits, not particularly related to the adjustment to aging.

- "Enjoyment of food" was found to be the primary factor to influence a food selection; "nutritious and healthful" was the next most important reason given.

- Price was given as a major consideration by only 11% of the sample. Annual income per person did influence weekly food expenditure, but neither income nor food cost had a significant effect on nutrient intake.

- Shopping practices were shaped, first by the ability to get to the store and second by the quality and type of food available.

Nutrient distribution over three meals per day were compared in families of all ages and older persons, all living at the poverty level (Guthrie et al., 1972).

- Older persons have a greater proportion of the nutrients at breakfast.
- The pattern of food consumption of older persons was similar to that of all ages.
- Snacks made up only 1/2 of their total intake as compared with families of all ages.
- Nutritional intake was not found to be influenced significantly by sex, education, self-ratings of health, dental health, or dietary restrictions.

Contrary to what is generally believed are the data from one study carried out by the National Analysts of Philadelphia for the United States Food and Drug Administration (Schneider and Hesla, 1973). The task was to investigate the nature and prevalence of health "fallacies, or questionable beliefs and practices." An extensive questionnaire was used to interview an American adult population. The results are hopeful if not typical.

- Older people are less likely than other adults to hold misconceptions about dietary adequacy and nutrient requirements.
- Forty-three percent never used vitamins or related products.
- Over one-half of those who used vitamins and tonics did so with medical advice.
- Vitamin users have a greater tendency for self-medication.
- Health food usage increases with increasing income and education.
- People with higher incomes are more weight-concerned and more likely to have received diets from a health professional.

In the examination of food patterns of older persons (202 men and 257 women) from the North Central region of the United States, many of the meals fell short of the goals suggested in the U.S. Department of Agriculture's GUIDE FOR OLDER FOLKS (Pao, 1971). Snacks were prevalent, some meat and many cereals were consumed, but vegetables, citrus fruits, and mineral-rich dairy products were used in only significant amounts.

An interesting inquiry into the food concerns of older persons has been conducted by the National Retired Teachers Association and the American Association of Retired Persons. Dr. Thomas Elwood, Coordinator of the Associations' health and education affairs carried out a study over a three-month period. The compilation served as a "profile of the concerns of this age group" (Elwood 1975). About 3,800 attended the health education program and asked a "total of 370 questions pertaining to nutrition" providing a valuable guide to educators and food industrialists alike:

- "Dieting is a concept with which they have some familiarity." Questions were concerned with the adequacy of fad diets; calories; "proper diet;" efficacy of artificial sweeteners: the dangers of sugar; nature, source, and means of control for cholesterol; how and where could they find a reliable source of information.

- These persons had real concern about the nature of food, food preparation and food intake. Questions emphasized the comparison of vitamin value in canned, fresh and frozen foods; changes in food quality upon cooking; proportions of protein essential; what kinds of protein; and meal patterns (6 meals versus 2 or 3).

- The connection between nutrition and health is generally accepted. Questions in this area were focused on the role of foods in causing disease, in the aggravation or amelioration of disease; does everyone need same amount of vitamin supplements?; what can vitamins C and E really do?; "health foods" and the regulation of "health food" stores.

For these older, mobile persons in the community (the majority), their involvement with body and self appears to be reflected in their marked interest in food. In spite of reduced incomes and other personal and status losses, many older persons indulge in costly dietary supplements (Elwood, 1975). With the "health" and "longer life" that some food advertising promises, this is an expected consequence.

Another investigation, carried out from February to December 1973 in Tennessee, looked particularly at the relationship between lifestyle and dietary inadequacy (Todhunder, 1976). The sample of 529 individuals 60 years and over were noninstitutionalized persons in middle Tennessee, males and females, blacks and whites, of different educational socio-economic backgrounds and living conditions from both rural and urban areas. Their beliefs about food and health provide an interesting mix of folklore and fact:

"Good for health" foods

all foods — 14% black males and females, white males; 5% white females

vegetables — named more often than any other food by both races and sexes; belief was consistent with practice.

"Bad for health" foods

pork — mentioned more frequently

food high in fat or fried — named by more than 10% of each subgroup most frequently by black males — 20%

sweets (desserts and candies) — 10% of participants

Their own diet

90% believed it was good and that food affected the way they felt.

84% of each subgroup said they had a good appetite for meals.

Willingness to try new foods

60% of each subgroup were willing. About 70% of subgroups had made some changes in food habits, mostly in recent years because of health, aloneness, beliefs, and a few for financial reasons.

Most important factor at mealtime

companionship	41% of white females
	34% of white males
	27% of black males
	25% of black females

food you like, and the way it is cooked	30% white females 36% black females

Favorite foods and most disliked foods

favorite

meat (mentioned most frequently)	beef 37% chicken 24% pork 10%
green beans	32%
greens	25%
potatoes	16%

disliked

disliked no foods	15%
cottage cheese	13% (most frequent)
many others mentioned	

Taste most frequently mentioned as reason for dislike.

Vegetables disliked because of texture or 'they disagree with me.'

Preferences

fresh produce	preferred by all subgroups

but canned food used by 85%
frozen foods used less frequently by blacks

Patterns

(1) Between-meal eating or snacking is a regular practice of only 37% of total group. The kind of food is predominantly protein-rich foods or dairy products; beverages infrequent.

(2) Comparatively few meals are eaten away from home, least often by black women.

(3) Breakfast is eaten regularly by over 90% of the group, eaten at home and was the favorite meal for more than one-third of each subgroup.

(4) The use of vitamin or mineral supplements was comparatively low; in about 15% of white males and females, almost negligible among blacks.

(5) More than 50% of the total group had a favorable attitude towards the need for food, did not economize by reducing expenditure. More blacks

than whites economize on food, the black female is the most disadvantaged. Meat was the first food to be cut down or out.

A large number of the subjects had nutrient intakes of less than two-thirds of the 1974 RDAs in spite of an overall positive attitude toward food, eating, and health. These persons exhibited noticeably little faddism, an openness to new foods and a necessity to alter food habits. Their responses to questions about food choice, meal patterns and beliefs lead to the tentative conclusion that economic capacity does play a significant role in dietary adequacy, contrary to the findings in the South Minneapolis housing development mentioned earlier (Noble, 1969). It appeared to limit both food choice and serving size (Todhunter, 1976).

No one study stands for all older persons in eating patterns, beliefs and practices, nor in food-related problems. But, there are some persuasive notions that appear frequently in the literature.

1. Older persons tend to increase carbohydrate intake, with a significant increase of refined sugars at the expense of the more nutritious carbohydrates, e.g. cereals. This is no doubt true because most of the carbohydrates (cakes, cereals, breads) are easier to chew, more palatable, and cost less than proteins, fats or fruits.

2. Subclinical malnutrition is more prevalent than heretofore considered. Exact nutritional requirements for older persons are still difficult to define, but generally the research indicates that malnutrition among older persons exists in different forms: overt, subclinical (requiring biochemical tests for detection) and marginal (observable only during or after a period of stress).

   Marginal malnutrition may contribute to increased vulnerability to disease and exaggerates the decline in homeostasis.

3. A high proportion of the subjects eat a diet deficient in one or more nutrients.

4. It is difficult to create a well balanced intake on a lower caloric intake (below 1800 calories) commensurate with

a significantly reduced level of physical activity. Generally, low-caloric diets may be characterized by deficient protein intake as well.

5. A high proportion of older persons eat institution-like food and a decreased amount of fresh food, such as raw vegetables, fruit or fruit juices.

6. It is not true that all necessary vitamins and nutrients are generally in ample supply in the diets of the majority of older persons. Calcium and iron are most frequently noted as deficient minerals. Calcium because of the reduction in milk and milk product intake and iron because of the decline in the diet of meat, fish and eggs. Vitamin C and the vitamin B-complex are most frequently in low or deficient amounts.

7. Most older persons show a tendency to take the greater proportion of nutrients at the breakfast meal. There may be important benefits from more careful planning to include maximum nutrients compatible with taste, income, and digestibility for this meal.

8. Diets of homemakers 55-74 years old were more adequate than those of older women (Le Bovit, 1965).

9. Although large numbers of older persons (in the studies examined) know about balanced diets, knowledge of basic food sources and functions is limited (Roundtree and Tinklin, 1975). Therefore, there is a substantial need for accurate nutrition information and education to motivate older persons to learn more about food, as well as for assistance in using new knowledge. Practices, however, were frequently not related to knowledge in the available studies.

10. Most older persons walk to the store and shop at a particular store because of closeness.

11. Eating is considered a social as well as a physiological function. Within groups of older poor, social isolation contributes to the lack of interest in foods and to dietary inadequacy.

Theories of Aging

7

Aging has been identified in a variety of ways — various disciplinary perspectives using different criteria. One of the most characteristic of all the processes of aging relates to the gradual decline of homeostatic capacity. Aging may then be considered a progressive, though gradual loss of adaptive capacity throughout the lifespan. Further, it may be said, this changing adaptive capability becomes most frequently observable in the middle and later years. There follows a decreased expectation of life with time, decreased viability and an increased vulnerability to disease and the force of mortality.

Over the last 20 years or so, theories and data about the "mechanisms of aging" have proliferated beyond the descriptive phase to the molecular bases for physiological activities. There is agreement among researchers only about the complexity of aging processes. In any number of the theories still with support, it is difficult to establish a simple, direct relationship between cause and effect. Without clear causality or mechanism, therapies in use (and proposed) for slowing the rate of aging are minimal in their effect and based primarily on suggestive data.

Some observers continue to see aging as a deficiency disease awaiting some replacement therapy. Others see changes with time as normal deterioration of function, inevitable and tolerable. Examples of involutional degeneration and death are found within normal development — generally clearly marked and predictable at specific times in the life-span e.g. the placenta during gestation, deciduous teeth and baby fat tissue in childhood and the ovaries after five decades or so.

AGING, THE RATE OF CHANGE AND ALL THE SPECIFIC ALTERATIONS RESULT FROM THE FALTERING AND RUNNING OUT OF A GENETIC PROGRAM.

That the genetic endowment plays a central role in aging is inescapable. One needs only to list the characteristic, species-specific mean and maximum lifespan of most living systems (Comfort, 1964; Rockstein, 1972) and the data from studies of monozygotic and dizygotic twins (Kallman and Jarvick, 1959).

The major work of Dr. Leonard Hayflick (1970) has demonstrated that cells in culture have a limited lifespan, also characteristic of the species. The immortality of human cells (as distinguished from the aging of the human organism) which was projected from the early work of Dr. Alexis Carrel (1921) with fibroblasts of the chick — is no longer a viable concept. Embryonic cells in culture reach a limit of 50± 10 population doublings. Moreover, this doubling capacity decreases with age, since cells from adult humans stop after about 20 doublings.

Dr. George Martin and colleagues (1970) confirmed and extended Dr. Hayflick's findings. Skin cells were cultured from arms of 100 subjects from fetal to 90 years, and demonstrated a decrease of 0.2 population doubling per year of donor life. Hayflick (1975) however, feels it is unlikely that animals age because one or more important cell populations lose their proliferative capacity. He maintains that — it is more probable that the metabolic changes which develop in the third phase, (before cessation of doubling and death) are more central and lead to the aberrations in structure and function.

THE ERROR THEORY OF AGING (MOLECULAR, ALSO INVOLVED WITH GENETIC SUBSTANCES)

The genetic apparatus may not include a particular program for aging but may with time, lose accurate and reliable information coded in the DNA and RNA. Loss of information may be due to random events which lead to cellular dysfunction, cessation of physiological activities and aging.

Alterations in chromosomal material, not necessarily mutations in DNA, are transmitted to RNA which translates the coded information into synthesis of protein and therefore enzymes. If the degree of alteration is such, that a number of defective or inactive enzymes are produced, this process could proceed to a point at which appropriate synthesis is no longer sufficient to compensate for the degree of consequent dysfunction. This reduces metabolic efficiency and interferes with the capacity for repair. Cell dysfunction and death become more frequent and with time and unmet demands of daily living — death of the organism occurs (Orgell, 1973).

AGING A RESULT OF DIFFERENT CHANGES IN NUCLEIC ACIDS: OTHER GENETIC CONCEPTS

Particular aspects of the genome have been investigated to provide clues for the explanation of different lifespans. It has been suggested that the degree of redundancy ratio in genes transcribing m RNA is the significant variable. Cutler (1974) found no definitive correlation between reiterated nucleotide sequence and aging rates, but redundancy ratio was suggestive. 1.3, 1.5, 2.1 found in the mouse, cow and human.

- Strehler (1967) has championed the notion that a sequential "turning off" of genes is responsible for aging.

- Burnett (1974) identified the immune system as central to aging, related to random mutations of DNA initiated in the thymus gland.

Data to support "aging as due to an accumulation of errors in DNA and protein synthesis" is equivocal (Moment, 1975).

- Some proteins have been identified with very low level changes.
- Collagen in tendons of old animals, though quite different from that in young animals is very similar to collagen of young when freshly synthesized (Hruza and Hlavachova, 1963).
- Though chromosomal aberrations increase in rat liver with time, liver regeneration still occurs (Crowley and Curtis, 1963). In the early stages of regeneration, RNA is typically fetal and with time becomes more like the adult.
- Therefore, genes, inactive for even an extended time in the lifespan of animals, are evidently not so altered, since they function well when called upon in regeneration.

AGING RESULTS FROM SOMATIC MUTATION.

This theory as the primary cause of aging has few supporters today. The belief that aging 'hits' are dominant is based on the work of Lamb and Maynard-Smith (1964), and Harris (1971) that concluded the effect of ionizing radiation on cells is in keeping with the assumption that radiation injury is dominant.

- However, such hits would be critical only if there was no repair capacity in the cell. Most cells do have a system of repair enzymes for DNA injury; endo-nuclease, repair polymerase and ligase (Sinex, 1974).
- Radiation studies of Curtis (1968) were used as support for the theory. Radiation damage increased tumor development and led to early death, rather than altered the rate of aging. This was supported by

the lack of differences in age-related physiological deterioration in the survivors of the atomic disaster of Nagasaki and Hiroshima (Hollingsworth et al., 1962). Radiation increased cancer incidence and premature death. Since radiation is a potent mutagen — yet it failed to increase the rate of aging — the usefulness of the somatic theory for aging is questionable.

MOST SINGULAR FACTOR IN AGING IS THE PROGRESSIVE, INTERMOLECULAR CROSS-LINKAGE OF COLLAGEN.

For proponents of this theory, collagen may also serve as a model for similar alterations and consequences in other proteins — reticulin, elastin and structural proteins of basement membranes. These changes are primarily applicable to the noncellular (intercellular) material of the body. The theory's rationale rests on the changes with time in collagen, the most abundant body protein (25-30%), and one of the 4 major constituents of connective tissue. In favor of widespread influences of collagen structure and function in aging is its ubiquity: in and around walls of blood vessels and around cells; muscle contracts and relaxes in a collagen-containing matrix; the exchange of substances between blood vessel and cell takes place in the intercellular tissue with collagen as a major constituent.

Apparent consequences of progressive cross-linking does appear throughout the body and interfere with:

- flexibility of muscle fibers with resultant decreased mobility,
- efficiency of cardiac muscle contraction in transmission of contractile force in large arteries (known to be more rigid),
- movement in intercellular space (decrease in profusion rate of organs),
- tissue oxygenation, which is reduced and leads to ischemia probably resulting from permeability changes which in turn leads to the trapping of lipids,

glycoproteins and minerals. With time, inflammation and lesions of atherosclerosis develop,

Result in:

- increased peripheral vascular resistance with resultant hypertension,
- impaired passage of gases, nutrients, metabolites, hormones, antibodies and accumulated toxins could explain increasing vulnerability to injuries, insult and heightened susceptibility to fatal disease,
- connective tissue alterations leading to hypoxia which may contribute to neoplasia.

It is clear that collagen changes and cross linking of other large molecules accompany age — it is not possible with data available however to specify cause and effect.

CHANGES IN IMMUNE FUNCTION, AUTOIMMUNITY, MAJOR FACTORS IN AGING

As defined by Walford (1969) the theory states that autoimmunity (and the autoantibodies) are primary determinants in cell dysfunctions which culminate in aging or cell death. There is widespread agreement with the working hypothesis "the fall in immune function predisposes in individual to illness" (Makinodan, 1975).

- Immune functions do reach a maximum in young adults and decline with age.
- Cancer and autoimmune diseases increase with age and appear associated with immune deficiency.
- Autoantibodies do carry out a necessary physiological function as well, by the initiation of phagocytosis of damaged cells by macrophages. It becomes important to discriminate between such 'physiologic' autoantibodies and 'pathologic' autoantibodies (Kay and Makinodan, 1976)
- Studies are still in progress to determine whether the diseases undermine immune capacity, or the fall in immune function predisposes the person to disease.

- Adler (1975) has provided evidence that one activity of T cells, (lymphocytes of thymus origin) decreases with age faster than does similar activity of B cells (lymphocytes of bone origin).
- Some suggest that antigens of the cell interior, normally protected, are exposed and recognized as foreign, possibly as a result of viral infection.
- Walford suggests loss of control of tolerance for self may cause an increase in autoimmune reactions and consequent aging.

FREE RADICALS (HIGHLY REACTIVE CELLULAR COMPONENTS) CAN ALTER OTHER IMPORTANT MO- LECULES CREATING MALFUNCTION OR DYSFUNC- TION THAT ACCUMULATE DURING THE LIFESPAN (HARMAN, 1971).

- This damage may occur in nuclear genetic materials, as in somatic mutations (Brooks et al., 1973) or in cytoplasm, particularly membrane surfaces and control molecules (Packer et al., 1967).
- Genic redundancy would appear to repair the chromosomal aberrations that develop.
- Data have been published to support the idea that "free-radical induced peroxidation of unsaturated fatty acids in organelle membranes and surface *in vivo* is a major determinant of biological aging" (Gordon, 1974).

1. It appears that free radical formation and consequent pathology *in vivo* are real events in aging; significance of these events to biological aging is not yet clear.
2. There is controversy about the use of *in vitro* findings since there is inadequate evidence for free radical effects on unsaturated lipids in living state (Green, 1972).
3. But new evidence has demonstrated the presence of lipid peroxidation products in phospholipid fraction of fresh human plasma (Di Luzio, 1973).

4. Tappel (1973) has demonstrated the presence of a fat derivative (age pigment) which increases with age in testes, heart and brain.

- There are many cellular changes that are found in aging organisms such as enhanced permeability, increased variability in the structure and function of mitochondria and microsomes, altered facilitated transport and the accumulation of lipid peroxidation products in cells and body fluids.

The major sites for free radical damage are biological membranes which are characterized by high concentration of unsaturated lipids. Included are mitochondria, microsomes and also free ribosomes and the cell surface. It is not difficult to conceive of widespread damage in many systems with a number of functional aberrations. The use of antioxidant drugs and vitamins inhibit and/or repair the lipid peroxidative damage and extend the life of experimental animals (Harman, 1968 a,b).

THERE ARE OTHER THEORETICAL APPROACHES TO AGING WHICH RELATE TO THE SIGNIFICANCE OF THE MAINTENANCE OF HOMEOSTASIS INVOLVING THE ENDOCRINE AND NERVOUS SYSTEMS.

If, as stated earlier, decreasing capacity for homeostasis is one of the most characteristic changes with time — then data and theories about aging of these two systems may come closer to the primary causes of aging than any of the others discussed earlier.

- Sacher (1968) states that the investigation of the coordinating neuroendocrine systems in development and aging is basic. The doubling of the human lifespan within the past two million years is surely related to brain development — its role in aging is inevitable, if not immediately obvious. He perceives a correlation with brain size and longevity.

- Sites of homeostatic control in the neuroendocrine system (such as the hypothalamus) are clearly implicated in changes through the lifespan.

(1) The reactivation of ovarian cycles in post oestrus female rats was achieved by electrical stimulation of the hypothalamus (Clemens et al., 1969).

(2) Livers of old mice have a decreased ability to synthesize the enzyme, tyrosine aminotransferase; an injection of hormones restored some of the earlier capacity (Finch, 1973).

In both of the reported instances, the age-related change was in the integrating tissues; in the first demonstrated by an inadequate message from the hypothalamus, in the second the decreased responsivity of a gland to neuronal stimulus.

- Pacemaker cells or organs represent another major concept

(1) Dilman (1971), in what he projects as "death clocks," suggests that "the genetic program for development and aging is a gradual elevation of the threshold of sensitivity of the hypothalamus to feedback suppression."

(2) Everitt (1973) has suggested the pacemaker is in the hypothalamus.

(3) Finch (1974) has continued to explore roles and metabolism of catecholamines in the hypothalamus as potential chemical evidence of age changes.

THOUGH NOT CONSIDERED A THEORY, ONE OF THE MOST PROMISING INVESTIGATIONS HAS BEEN THE CONTRIBUTION OF DIET TO THE RATE OF AGING.

Nutrition has become a tool in the attempts to test some of the foregoing hypotheses. There remains the hidden hope that some nutritional intervention could "stay" the rate of aging. For many, the management of food may be the magic for everlasting youth and vigor.

It all began with McCay and colleagues (1935) who demonstrated that a reduced caloric diet for very young rats increased the lifespan. This has been pursued by

1. Miller and Payne (1968) increased rats' lifespan 28% with a high-protein diet during the first 4 months of postnatal life, and a very low protein diet thereafter.

2. Ross and Bras (1974) have shown that time of onset of various age-related diseases in rats can be delayed by diet. Death, which is ordinarily caused by lung or kidney diseases in the rats under study is therefore also delayed. The diet restrictions have left some of the rats looking sickly; others healthy, but sterile, and some healthy, but undersized. Up to this point, these diets have not been tried with primates. Such studies would provide additional insight to the potential for human implementation.

Manipulation of the diet was also attempted with other targets in mind to retard aging:

1. Slowing the maturation of the immune response which appears to be at a low level in young animals was attempted by Walford and Liu (1973). They hypothesize that suppression of immunity in early life may delay the development of autoantibodies during aging.

2. The use of unsaturated fats in the diet would influence aging (similarity in structure of free radical substance and unsaturated fats) by slowing the rate of degradation (Walford, 1971).

   • The mean lifespan of the female mice was significantly decreased.

   • Increase in mortality from mammary cancer which suggests that lipid free radicals may increase the carcinogenicity of the tumor agent.

   • Increase in dietary vitamin E minimizes the effect.

It was concluded by Harman (1972) that degradative changes in biological systems may be developed in part by endogenous free radical reactions as observed in:

1. oxidative changes in collagen, elastin and chromosomal material

2. mucopolysaccharide oxidative degradation

3. oxidative polymerization involving lipids and proteins

leading to accumulation of age pigments.

Data suggest that the use of one or more free radical inhibitors in a nutritionally adequate diet may increase the average age of death. Projected to the human lifespan, there is an expected increase of average age at death of 7 or more years.

New technology and more molecular data will continue to pursue the mechanisms of aging. Increasingly, researchers do not expect to find *one primary* cause of aging. Changes with time would appear to be multifactorial. Greater focus has come to rest on testable theses in the physiology of the whole organism. Investigation of the interacting systems (hormonal and neuronal) and their physiological goal — homeostasis — would appear likely to yield worthwhile information. Many of the degenerative diseases associated with age have also proven to be susceptible (within limits) to nutritional intervention. The definitive role established for nutrition in early and later growth, development and maintenance (particularly for the nervous system) and the research of Harman (1968 a,b, 1972) Ross (1972) and McCay (1935, 1955) suggest a significant therapeutic and possible preventive function for nutrition in relation to aging.

$\mathcal{S}$ummation 8

SUMMARY

A number of the pertinent questions related to nutrition and age have been addressed, and present similar as well as contradictory data. Admittedly, some issues are less well-defined and the critical studies are not completed or, in fact, designed. The exponential increase in the last three years of research reports and review articles related to nutrition and aging is encouraging. Although we may still lack for reasonable, validated answers to pressing issues, the interest and talent represented maximize (at the very least) the probability for posing the purposeful questions.

The human body needs 50 or more nutrients from which to provide energy and metabolites. There is a continuing though changing requirement all through the lifespan for the kind of food intake that provides as many of these nutrients as possible for the maintenance of optimum physiology and physique. In spite of currently discrepant data, the increase in investigative activity holds promise.

General concepts in relation to food at any age relate as well to older persons: to maintain homeostasis, to prevent structural loss, to improve handling of all types of stress and to promote mental and physical vigor. Food has been variously classified in studies, not always supported with reproducible data from investigations with appropriate controls. Persons other than scientists also perceive food as fulfilling a number of roles; some magic and others more mundane, but essential.

therapy: in instances of identified deficiencies (e.g. mineral or vitamin deficiency, protein, caloric or fatty acid deficiencies)

a preventive measure: *in utero* diet for the benefit of fetus and infant

source of metabolites/energy: for maintenance of tissue structure and function

a specific tool: in the retardation of aging (e.g. yogurt; apricot extract; antioxidant vitamins C and E).

a symbol: of affection and concern from others (positive); as a substitute for living and life satisfaction (negative)

finally, a cure-all: mama's chicken soup, herb tea.

My own evaluation of changing requirements with age agrees with a statement by Tunbridge (1961) after he reviewed the literature on diet and aging: "There was sufficient evidence to confirm the belief of the ancients — that an optimum diet for older persons is different from that of the young adult." Further noted, but frequently ignored in practice, is the reality that the diet for the well older person is often not appropriate for the chronically or acutely-ill older person.

In spite of the Tunbridge view stated 16 years ago, careful longitudinal studies concerning nutritional needs of the later years are few and limited in approach. The literature in the 1960's continued to emphasize that nutritional needs of the elderly are very similar to the needs of other adults (Morgan, 1962; Stare, 1962; Watkin, 1968). Finally, Taylor (1973 a,b) advised that older persons should have a higher intake of protein-rich and protective foods.

Malnutrition, as overeating, is a serious problem in the middle and early older years (the "young old"). This country has been witness to a significant change in dietary patterns away from raw fruits, vegetables, dairy products and proteins of meat origin. For too many, today's diet is still high in cholesterol and other lipids, sugar, and refined grains — almost 20% refined sugar and 45% fat. These nutrients have been implicated in tooth decay, atherosclerosis, obesity, diabetes and heart disease.

A decrease in vascular mortality has taken place in the United States from 1950-1975[1]. By 1975 the decline in cardiovascular deaths exceeded the noncardiovascular by 60%. This may be part of the sign that Americans are becoming sensitive to the recommendations of the American Heart Association (begun in 1964) to limit dietary intake of saturated fats and cholesterol (Walker, 1977). Preliminary data from the National Center for Health Statistics demonstrate an even lower death from ischemic heart disease in the first half of 1976 than in first half of 1975.[2] Other aspects of the life style, nevertheless, are no doubt involved e.g. reduction in smoking, physical fitness programs. Nevertheless the diminution of per capita consumption (since 1964) in animal fats, oils, butter, liquid milk, cream and eggs and the associated increase in consumption of vegetable fats and oils is persuasive and suggests a correlation (Walker, 1977).

The "westernized" diet described also tends to lack bulk, and the inferential, descriptive evidence connects this lack to the development of diverticular disease and malignancy. Some empirical, experimental data appear to confirm these tentative conclusions, but additional studies are essential to resolve still contradictory data.

On the basis of the materials and studies examined, a serious yet generally neglected issue is touched on repeatedly — the widespread subacute or subclinical malnutrition that appears to exist among persons over 55 years of age. Even a quick glance at the data accumulated for the Ten-State Survey (1968-70) leads one to believe that older persons

---

[1]National Heart, Lung, and Blood Institutes 'Fact Book for Fiscal Year 1976 DHEW Publication #77-1172 Washington, D.C. Government Printing Office, 1976, p.14.

[2]*Monthly Vital Statistics Vol. 26* (7), September 24, 1976

often have a low intake of some important regulatory nutrients (vitamins and minerals) frequently unsatisfactory general nutriture and deficiency. Specific nutrients include calcium, iron, magnesium vitamins A, C, thiamin, niacin and especially folic acid.

Frank protein deficiency, as a result of low dietary intake, is not seen as often in the reported studies as had been expected. Low serum proteins and low amino acids are more common — no doubt because in the reduced caloric intake, (with low carbohydrate, fat and protein) the available reduced protein has been used for energy production.

There are suggestions in the literature (Hazzard, 1976; Inoye, 1975) that a more careful appraisal of the caloric needs of older persons must take place to avoid the general advice of 'eat less.' It may be that most older persons (ambulatory and in the community; ill and hospitalized and/or in significant stress) are in greater caloric need than heretofore thought. Efficiency for work decreases with time, protein synthesis diminishes and older persons will probably lose weight without effort as they grow older still (Hazzard, 1976).[3]

Continued use of the current RDAs, which serve for many studies as reference for the calculation of nutritional adequacy, concerns me. These values, estimated to exceed the requirements for most persons, and developed with the "reference" person (healthy, young, active) as the base, do not relate to the individuality and heightened differences among older persons. These were meant as guides (Harper, 1975) and should be increased to cover the range of individual differences and situations. Harper[4] (1975) has said, "When in doubt, select higher alternative values because there is no evidence that small surplus of nutrients are harmful, whereas, small deficits over time lead eventually to depletion and deficiency." The 51+ years values for nutrients

---

[3]W.R. Hazzard. Communication to author. *Summary Opinion: Nutrition in the Aged.*

[4]Chairman of Committee on Dietary Allowances of Food and Nutrition Board, 1974 National Research Council, National Academy of Sciences.

do not consider the differentiation that occurs within such a large group. There is a need to carefully calculate a series of RDA values that will accommodate information now available about aging and older persons.

While malnutrition among older persons has no single causal factor, significant in subclinical malnutrition may be the multiple kinds of stress that middleaged and older persons experience in Western society. The older person faces significant changes in life style: in life space, in loss of friends or spouse, in work status, in economic wherewithal, in isolation — as well as in the gradual changes in physical capacity and function. Early work suggests that life changes alone may be important gerontological stress factors. Rahe et al., (1967) found that there was a 75% correlation between the number of life change units on a "Social Readjustment Rating Scale" (e.g., death of a spouse, retirement, divorce, etc.), and the seriousness of illness within the following year. Studies to develop positive, adaptive mechanisms to stress (biofeedback, exercise) could reduce the potential pathogenic effect of stress.

Nutrition provides the raw materials for energy and synthesis. Illness leads in a circular fashion to poorer nutrition, which further decreases the immune competence necessary to weather illness and results in exacerbation and/or continuation of illness. With that as a background, the consideration of the "synergistic" effects of malnutrition and stress (Scrimshaw, 1964, 1966) in the older person becomes an area of inquiry that requires urgent attention.

There is sufficient evidence in the literature, (though not related primarily to the older years) for stress-induced loss of homeostatic balance in nitrogen, calcium, vitamin C, and some of the B complex vitamins. It is reasonable that an even more acute imbalance of many nutrients would be measurable among older persons who are already in low nutritional status. Their physiological capacities and homeostatic responses are in gradual decline. Data do exist that attest to cellular death (and finally tissue necrosis) with sufficient micronutrient imbalance over an extended period. Imposed on the emotional, and other environmental stress referred to earlier, illness becomes still another critical player in the synergy.

In view of these realities of aging, as we know them today, it can be misleading to state that the nutritional needs of older persons are little different from other adults. With the described, built-in demands for stress response, select nutrients would appear to be essential in greater amounts on a regular, rather than 'one-time,' basis with appropriate regard for the dangers of excessive intake of particular nutrients and calories. However, Schlenker maintains that "the only nutrient requirement which does appear to change is the need for calories" (1976)[5]. On the other hand, she cautions that the determination of nutritional status of older persons cannot be based on any single factor and must include biochemical, clinical as well as dietary measurements. Alfin-Slater (1976)[6] sees advantages in a changing pattern of meals per day for older persons, "the 'five-snack' system may be best nutritionally — as well as decreasing the likelihood of 'indigestion' and spacing and increasing the number of the days' pleasurable events."

Benefits of good nutrition take time, and cannot be evaluated in a week or a month(s). Short term studies may provide negative or equivocal data, at best clues for the long term approach. Evidence has been presented (Schlenker, 1973; Mayer, 1974; Watkin, 1973) that nutritional adequacy in early life is related to health and well being in later life. However, the older years are not too late for the reestablishment of adequate nutrition, attested to by the countless examples in the foregoing pages.

RESEARCH PRIORITIES

1. An important, albeit laborious step would be both cross-sectional and longitudinal investigations to determine accurate nutrient intake and nutrient serum and/or tissue levels essential for older persons. This would enable the development of nomograms for reference and

[5]E. D. Schlenker. Communication to author. *Commentary* (on nutrition in the aged).

[6]Alfin-Slater, R.B. Communication to author. *Nutritional Patterns Appropriate to Well Elderly*.

research and practice. RDAs suitable for middle aged and older persons would then take care of themselves.

One of the the important areas to be carefully studied across the lifespan are the so called 'mild deficiencies,' essentially asymptomatic until some stress reveals the inadequacies.

Longitudinal studies could provide knowledge that would enable the identification of the sequence of changes in nutritional status throughout the lifespan that contribute to long life, free of debilitating disease. Particular information is necessary to differentiate diets for the ill/well elderly, for the invalid/active, for the 'young' and 'old' old. The 51+ group as identified in the RDA tables is far from homogeneous: sub-groups exist related to age, activity and pathology.

2. One of the attractive hypotheses in the delay of aging is underfeeding. Much remains to be done and tested beyond the excellent suggestive rat studies. Inquiries need to be designed to investigate the mental and physical consequences of undernutrition in the human.

3. Careful, rational biochemical and physiological analyses of vegetarian intake and its effect on health should be undertaken. There are indications in the literature that vegetarians may enjoy better health and are less at risk related to atherosclerosis, coronary heart disease and cancer. Some confusion of terms and diverse conclusions characterize the increasing references to the role of fiber in the prevention of cancer and heart disease. Recent studies point to a reduced risk of various concerns among Seventh Day Adventists (Phillips, 1975) and Mormons (Enstrom, 1975). It is inevitable that scientific observers will consider that some of this reduction may be related to abstention from tobacco and alcohol, which is true for most people of both religious groups. However, reduced mortality from gastrointestinal cancers cannot be due solely to nutritional factors, since some Adventists are lacto-ovo vegetarians, while the rest generally eat meat. Again, as with so much pathology, a plurality of influences including dietary ones must be examined.

4. There is insufficient evidence that older persons are significantly better off with the incorporation of large amounts of meat into the diet, or in fact with high protein. The high meat diets are reported to result at times in acidoses, in addition to the potential imbalance of the calcium/phosphate ratio. There are those who argue that with the decline in renal function accompanying age, increased protein over the recommended RDA intake (.6g of high quality protein/kg.) is a metabolic hazard, since any excess protein catabolized to urea must be excreted through less than efficient kidneys (Theuer, 1971)[7]. However, repeated reference to the need for high dietary protein to fight disease indicates that work remains to be done, examining the apparent connection between high protein intake and maintenance of immunocompetency.

5. Few specific references and research are available, but frequently allusions exist noting the significance of the interaction of nutrients, e.g. effect of carbohydrate intake in the etiology of lipidemia; protein-sparing role of carbohydrates, interaction among calcium, phosphorous and magnesium affecting absorption of each. This remains a relatively unexplored area.

6. The role of calcium, fluoride and hormonal therapy in osteoporosis is still in contention − e.g., despite the Bantu's low intake of calcium and almost completely vegetarian diet, there appears to be no osteoporosis. This may be due to the substantial calcium in many vegetables. However, white residents of South Africa with a high protein and high fat diet do exhibit slight acid-demineralization.

7. The real potential of diet therapy plus rehabilitation (exercise) to restore reduced body mass (muscle and bone) has not been pursued in organized research. This requires a commitment of time and energy for documentation so that new information can be effectively

---

[7]Report in *Dairy Council Digest Vol. 48*(1). Jan/Feb. 1977 p.3.

translated for use. Nathan Pritikin, (a nutrition scientist and director at the Longevity Research Institute in Santa Barbara) and Dr. David Blankenhorn at the University of Southern California have been experimenting with diet therapy and exercise (Isaacs, 1976). Pritikin is convinced of the effectiveness of his rigorous, fat-free diet and exercise regimens in the reversal of atherosclerosis and hypertension in his patients, and predicts 90% success. He reports that more than 70 people with the heart ailment, angina, have been cured, and patients set for coronary bypass surgery are no longer in need of the procedure. Blankenhorn (1976)[8] also reports that 9 out of 40 patients following a similar diet have also begun to recover. These studies provide positive but still only suggestive evidence. All that can now be said is that "atherosclerosis can be reversed in the human." (Blankenhorn, 1976). The reversibility of atherosclerosis, earlier thought to be irreversible once started, is the topic of an entire issue of Triangle (Gresham, 1976). Pritikin's regimens have been called "way-out, unscientific" by Dr. Peter Wood, Deputy director of the Heart Disease Program at Stanford University in Palo Alto, but Wood thinks Pritikin "is doing what has to be done. I wouldn't be the least bit surprised if all his claims turn out to be true."[9]

8. There is remarkably little in the research literature related to hydration, although dehydration is not uncommon among older persons. Water is easily overlooked as a major requirement. Yet its central importance is apparent as the medium for cellular reactions, and as part of the body's continual attempt to maintain salt and water balance in view of the progressive loss of tissue fluid with age.

9. Maturity-onset diabetes is most frequently classified as a disease, but critical questions remain. Perhaps we are

---

[8]Cited in Isaacs, 1976

[9]Reported in New West, Feb. 14, 1977 p.60.

now closer to clearer definition with necessary techniques in hand which may provide reasonable answers to the questions of glucose tolerance and insulin response with age. Does maturity-onset diabetes represent normal adaptation with age and changing systemic responsivity, or a disease entity?

10. Stress has been implicated for some time in the investigations of pathology — cardiovascular dysfunction, hypertension and atherosclerosis in the middle years. Stress among older persons is just beginning to be considered a variable with which to contend." Because of this, renewed interest has developed in the identification of personality types with characteristic response to stress.

11. Much remains to be learned concerning vitamin and megavitamin therapy for use with particular symptomology or as preventive treatment. Additional controlled investigations into the benefits and potential risks of this increasingly discussed approach may help to resolve on-going controversies and diverse data.

12. Indications in the literature suggest that acute nutritional deficiencies or prolonged subclinical malnutrition are associated with faulty or inefficient drug therapy, with disease and decreased immunocompetence. With hospitalization, institutionalization, and immobilization and/or the multitude of interacting factors — psychosocial factors, disease and malnutrition, the inability to adequately mount a defense to disease is inescapable. There are insufficient data to make a definitive judgement on the advisability of food supplements or food fortification. It makes sense for the basic and clinical investigators to cooperate with the food industry for the development of studies which will determine the effectiveness and safety of nutrient fortification and supplementation. This suggestion, as a priority, was raised also by a clinical investigator for whom the nutrition and health of older persons represent major concerns and expertise (Hazzard, 1976)[10].

---

[10] Hazzard, op cit.

13. It would appear necessary to launch a massive evaluation of the nutritional programs that have grown out of the national effort, The Nutritional Program for Older Americans (NPOA). Since August of 1973, 4500 meal service sites have been established. As of June 30, 1976 there were 845 additional projects with an average number of meals daily over 257,000. In Fall 1977, a 40% increase is expected,[11] but will still serve only a small percentage of all over 60 years of age. Careful documentation concerning the benefits and inadequacies of such programs related to nutritional status and health of older persons is not available.

14. As an important corollary, there is also a need for the study of the role of nutrition education for all health practitioners and the public at large to determine how attitudes and behaviors are changed.

CONCLUSION

The literature has moved, even in the last five years from overwhelmingly descriptive papers to the analytical. There is increasing incorporation of nutritional adequacy as a principle variable in the quality, and possibly the length, of life. It is clear that nutrition is one of major environmental factors in resistance to disease, tolerance to stress, and as a consequence, of possible significance in the extension of life beyond current life expectations.

The kind, quality, quantity, and timing of nutrient intake, as well as interactions of foods with physiology have been examined in this monograph. However, there is considerable evidence that the final disposition and usefulness of food relates to all aspects of living. To avoid the trap 'food alone is important,' the total appraisal of nutritional adequacy requires the consideration of many life-long influences, and the biochemical clinical physiology. However, for the focus of this work, attention to the affective, psychological, and a variety of sociological variables

---

[11]*Dairy Council Digest Vol. 48*(1) Jan/Feb. 1977 p.5.

has been minimal.

Nutrition is more than food, and perhaps more acutely so with older persons as life space diminishes and characteristics of daily living increasingly relate to deprivation. Significant are: motivation towards eating, customary and cultural attitudes and practices, general mental and physical health, isolation, availability of food, geography, transportation, economics, and education in the use of food.

It is encouraging to note that intervention potential in all these aforementioned areas is great. As suggested throughout these pages, intervention appears possible as well in many specific areas of deficiencies and pathologies.

Action for nutrition and aging could include nutritional education, nutrient supplements, food fortification, overall health assessment and caring. In order to be effective, (and not merely crisis-oriented), these activities should be part of a lifespan of 'nutrition for living.'

For now and the future, however, emphasis on 'nutrition for prevention' of subclinical and clinical malnutrition would suggest that the middle years are a priority target, in addition to the older years. For now, the diet of older persons, whether at home or in institutions, should be considered adequate only after a creaful reexamination of the commercial preparation of food, cooking of meals, daily nutrient intake, clinical and biochemical tests, and overall behavior. Any preventive or therapeutic approach demands attention to the whole person and the environment.

For now and for the future, the research must continue to test the inferred and suggest therapies to finally insure that a reasonable answer may be provided to the nutritional questions of clinicians, nutritionists, and older persons themselves — appropriate to the real individuals involved. Moreover, since the future will find middle aged and older persons greater in number, healthier, more active, and better educated, the scientists and clinicians must commit themselves to the design of investigations not only for the present, but for the foreseeable changes.

Particularly important in the continuity of knowledge and its application, is the support for a 'renaissance of nutritional science' in more institutions at all levels of learning. At present there are some excellent centers across the country, some in Food Sciences,[12] others in Nutrition[13], and some who have made the logical combination. The road to improved nutritional status for the young and the old has many steps, but one that has been missed is the presence of a widespread, respected, academic (teaching and research) area in nutrition. A dimension within nutrition that has been sorely lacking is the concentration of knowledge and effort in 'Nutrition through the Life Cycle.' As it stands, lay persons and most academicians must plow through mounds of opinion — much inexpert and faddist — and continue to want for order out of chaos.

The physicians and other allied health professionals who attend older persons, both in communities and institutions, must also suffer the ignorance of their own deficient education in nutrition and in aging. Those presently in the middle and later years are often the unhappy beneficiaries of these educational inadequacies. Vigorous, continuous emphasis from Dr. Robert Butler, Director of the National Institute on Aging, from members of the Gerontological Society and American Geriatrics Society to create a position in the curriculum for Geriatrics beyond the 'elective' route, is part of the changing educational environment. There have been increasingly positive activities in the medical schools within the past two years which will encourage the support of attention to nutrition and the lifespan.

There is other 'good news.' The significant growth within the past 5-8 years of the field of gerontology within institutions of higher learning has provided impetus to the very recent, excellent symposia and research undertakings on selected topics in nutrition and age. The literature within the past two years includes more scholarly reviews, and also nutrition bibliographies for educational purposes.[14,15]

Gerontology, health professionals, nutrition, and the nutritional status of older persons would appear to have reached an important crossroads — the threshold or

---

[12]Massachusetts Institute of Technology, Rutgers, Michigan State, University of California at Davis.

[13]Tulane University, Pennsylvania State, U.C. Berkeley, U.C. Davis, Cornell, Massachusetts Institute of Technology.

activation energy is available. The potential consequences of such a cooperative enterprise for health maintenance and improvement among the middle aged and older persons are meaningful for many sectors of the population: the lay person, the allied health practitioner, and governmental agencies. It is apparent that important studies remain to be carried out. Nevertheless, what information is available can be transmitted to those who need to know, so that nutritional practices for and by older persons may begin to wear the cloak of the 1970's. Changes can be instituted in thinking and practices, even as scientific investigations move to increase our new knowledge and sophistication.

[14]*Present Knowledge in Nutrition* 4th ed. the Nutrition Foundation, Inc. Wash. D.C. 1976.

[15]*Education in Nutrition for Physicians and Dentists, An Annotated Bibliography* the Nutrition Foundation, Inc. 1976.

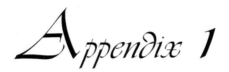

GLOSSARY

achlorhydria: absence of hydrochloric acid from the gastric juice.

adipocyte: a fat cell.

adiposity: a state of malnutrition in which excessive fat accumulation disturbs body functions; a condition in which body weight is about 20% or more above desirable weight.

anabolism: snythesis; processes by which simple substances are converted by living cells into more complex substances; includes chemical reactions nutrients undergo in their transformation and incorporation into body tissues, such as blood, enzymes, muscle and fat.

anorexia: pathological absence of hunger or appetite in spite of physiological need.

antibody: protein substance synthesized in response to the presence of antigens (substances usually foreign to the organism); function primarily to overcome toxicity of antigens.

arterial intima: the innermost coat of an artery; consists of endothelium and usually a thin subendothelial layer.

atherogenesis: formation of atheroma, fatty substances

which cause fatty degeneration of the inner layer of the arteries.

atheromatosis: the processes in which lesions of athero-sclerosis develop; collection of lipids in the walls (the intima and media) of the arteries.

autoimmunity: the condition in which antibodies are produced in response to the subject's own tissues, leads to tissue damage; may be identified by autoimmune antibodies and/or necrosed tissues, or other symptoms of autoimmune diseases.

basal metabolism or basal metabolitic rate (BMR): min-imum energy (food) needed to carry on body processes vital to life; measured by oxygen consumed and carbon dioxide released; basal metabolic rate is a measure of the 'idling speed' of cellular respiration, the minimum food and energy required to carry on body processes necessary to maintain life; a reflection of the activity of thyroid whose hormones are secreted at a relatively constant rate; can be measured by oxygen consumed and carbon dioxide released or by the PBI (protein bound iodine test) which measures the amount of iodine bound to protein in blood (as opposed to free); BMR varies with sex, age, hormones, health and nutritional status.

bolus: a soft mass of masticated food, a pliable ball of food rolled into shape by movement of tongue and saliva.

catabolism: the breakdown in the body of complex sub-stances into simpler ones, resulting in liberated energy (heat, electrical, mecanical); opposite of anabolism; catabolism and anabolism constitute metabolism.

catecholamines: hormones (epinephrine, norepinephrine and their precursor, dopamine) which share a common chemical stress, and are considered to be 'stress' hormones that enable mobilization of resources to meet emotional and physical changes; norepinephrene and dopamine, found in the brain also considered to be major neurotransmitters.

cecum: a blind pouch; the first part of the large intestine from which the appendix is suspended.

cheilosis: cracks and fissures at the corners of the mouth characteristic of riboflavin deficiency.

cholesterol: an alcohol lipid present in all animal fats and also synthesized by the body; circulates in the blood as lipoprotein (normal range from 150 to 250 mg/100ml); is presently considered by some researchers to be one of the substances related to high blood pressure, atheroma (hardening of the arteries), gallstones and other diseases.

colitis: acute or chronic inflammation of the colon or large bowel due to one or more causes.

colorectal cancer: cancer of the colon and rectum.

coronary occlusion: blockage of a coronary vessel usually by thrombosis and generally leading to infarction (necrotic changes due to obstruction of an end artery) of the myocardium; obstruction of flow of blood through an artery of the heart as the result of spasm of the vessel or the presence of a clot formed by coagulation of the blood or progressive atherosclerosis.

diverticula: a pouch or sac opening from a tubular or sacular organ, such as the gut or bladder.

diverticulitis: inflammatory condition of a civerticulum (a) characterized by vomiting, nausea, fever, abdominal tenderness, distention, pain and intestinal spasm; may eventually lead to intestinal obstruction or perforation, necessitating surgery.

dizygotic twins: fraternal twins; derived from two separate zygotes.

duodenum: first portion of the small intestine, extending from the pylorus to the jejunum.

edema: accumulation of excessive amount of fluid in cells, tissues, or serous cavities.

electrolyte: a substance that, in solution, conducts an electric current and ionizes into an electrically charged particle; examples: sodium ($Na+$), potassium ($K+$), Calcium ($Ca++$); electrolyte solutions such as body fluids.

endogenous: originating or coming from within or inside the cell or tissue.

endothellium: membrane that lines the closed cavities of the body such as the heart, blood vessels and the lymph vessels.

enzyme: organic compound, protein in nature, synthesized by living cells; accelerates metabolic reactions-hydrolases, oxidases, transferases, dehydrogenases, peptidases, etc.

essential amino acid: fundamental structural units of protein which cannot be synthesized by the body from materials readily available at a speed commensurate with the demands for normal growth; must therefore be supplied, preformed in the diet.

exogenous: coming from or originating from outside the body.

fibroblast: connective tissue cell; a spindle-shaped cell with a thin layer of cytoplasm and a large, oval, flattened nucleus; forms the fiberous tissues on the body.

flatulence: condition where gases are generated in the stomach or intestines.

follicular hyperkeratosis: skin changes due to severe vitamin A deficiency; rough, dry, scaly skin, the result of plugged sebaceous glands due to keratinized epithelium.

food and nutrition board: Food and Agriculture Organization (FAO); United Nations branch involved with adequate food supplies and nutrition, worldwide.

gastroenteritis: inflammation of the mucous membrane of both the stomach and intestine.

genome: a complete set of chromosomes (diploid number) derived from one parent, the haploid number of a gamete.

glucose: the 7 carbon sugar found in the blood; obtained by the hydrolysis of starch, sucrose, maltose, and lactose; a monosaccharide occurring in fruits and honey, dextrose, grape sugar, the metabolic breakdown of which generates energy in all cells; the blood glucose level is maintained homeostatically at a reasonably constant level (between 70 to 120 mg percent).

glossitis: inflammation of the tongue; may be a symptom of a gastrointestinal disorder or deficiency in one or more of the B complex vitamins.

glycogen: polysaccharide produced from glucose by the liver or the muscle; "animal" starch.

homeostasis: "constancy of the internal environment," the ability of the body to maintain balance of its physiochemical processes dependent on dynamic states of metabolism; physiological parameters under homeostatic control include: fluid and pH level, heart and pulse rates, and hormonal activities.

hormone: organic substance produced by an organ and discharged directly into the bloodstream for a specific regulatory action on other organs or tissues remote from its original source; generally manufactured by the endocrine glands; examples: insulin, thyroxine, and estrogens.

hyperadrenocorticism: excessive secretion of the adrenocortical hormones, usually cortisol.

hypercholesterolemia: condition marked by higher than normal levels of blood cholesterol.

hyperglycemia: increased glucose concentration in the blood above normal limits; may occur in the following conditions: diabetes mellitus due to lack of insulin; increased epinephrine secretion; following ingestion of a very high carbohydrate intake; hyperthyroidism due to increased hepatic glycogenolysis; increased intracranial pressure; administration of anesthetics such as ether, chloroform, and morphine and hyperpituitarism.

hyperlipidemia: nonspecific term that refers to an excess of fat in the blood.

hypertension: also called high blood pressure; elevation of blood pressure above normal.

hyperthyroidism: endocrine disorder caused by excessive secretion of the thyroid hormone; increases the rate of metabolic activity including nutrient breakdown; may be caused by a number of factors including drugs, hyperactivity of the thyroid gland or tumor; symptoms include thyroid enlargement, increased pulse rate, nervousness, muscle tremors and loss of weight, and there may also be protruding eyes.

hypertriglyceridemia: elevated triglyceride concentration in blood.

hyperuricemia: enhanced blood concentration of uric acid.

hypervitaminosis: vitamin toxicity; produced by excessive ingestion of fat soluble vitamins, especially A and D.

iatrogenic: related to or characterized by an abnormal state or condition produced by the physician or medicant in a patient by inadvertent or erroneous treatment.

insulin: a hormone secreted by the beta cells of the Islands of Langerhans of the pancreas; promotes utilization of glucose and lower blood sugar; lack of insulin leads to diabetes mellitus.

internal elastic lamina: a layer of elastic tissue of the tunica intima of arteries (see arterial intima).

in vitro: in the test tube, outside the living organism; referring to chemical reactions, fermentations, etc.

in vivo: in the living body; referring to vital biochemical processes as distinguished from those occurring in the test tube.

ischemic: local anemia due to mechanical or chemical obstruction (mainly arterial narrowing) to the blood supply; deficiency of the blood in a body part, due to functional constriction or actual obstruction of a vessel.

ischemic heart disease: heart disease relating to or due to ischemia.

isotonic: refers to a solution, having the same tension or pressure particularly in relation to body tissues, example; the importance of body fluids or introduced solution having the same toxicity as red blood cells.

kilocalorie (kcalorie): the amount of heat required to raise 1000 grams of water one degree centigrade; used in nutrition, also known as the large calorie (C or Calorie).

lipids: an inclusive term for fats and fat-like substances, characterized by the presence of one or more fatty acids; including fats, cholesterol, lecithins, phospholipids, and similar substances, which do not mix readily with water.

lumen: cavity or channel within a tubular organ, such as in an artery, vein, or intestine.

megaloblastic anemia: type of anemia characterized by an increased level of megaloblasts, primitive nucleated red blood cells much larger than the mature normal erythrocytes; the megaloblastic anemias respond readily to folic acid therapy and an adequate diet.

metabolism: physical and chemical changes occurring within the organism; includes synthesis of biologic materials and breakdown of substances to yield energy; includes both anabolism and catabolism.

micelle: water-soluble microscopic particles capable of penetrating the mucosal membrane; formed when free fatty acids, monoglycerides, some diglycerides and triglycerides and cholesterol are complexed with bile salts.

microsome: part of the cell that is composed of the ribosomes and endoplasmic reticulum.

mitochondria: cell organelle in which oxidative respiration, the most efficient energy (ATP) producing reactions of the cell take place, site for the Krebs cycle and electron transfer system.

monozygotic twins: type of twins resulting from a single fertilized ovum that at an early stage of development becomes separated into independently growing cell aggregates giving rise to two individuals of the same sex and identical genetic constitution; also called (enzygotic), identical twins.

neoplasia: process resulting in formation of new and abnormal growth, such as a tumor.

neuron: nerve cell consisting of the nerve cell body and its various processes; the dendrites, axon, and arborized ending.

neurotransmitter: a chemical secreted at the nerve ending and transmitting impulses to another sensory or motor end plate.

nomogram: a graph of two known values from which a third can be determined; used to calculate the surface area of the body from its height and weight.

occult bleeding: concealed hemorrhaging; blood in the feces in amounts too small to be seen but detectable by chemical tests.

organelle: an anatomically and functionally specialized part of a tissue cell.

osteomalacia: a manifestation of calcium deficit in which bones lose their calcium, phosphorous and other electrolytes, become soft and pliable, causing a shrinkage in height.

osteoporosis: a disease in which chemical composition of the bone remains unchanged (normal), but a disorder in which both mineral and supporting matrix are lost from the bone becoming thinner, lighter and more porous.

oxidation: :a process by which oxygen is added to a molecule or hydrogens and electrons are removed, and energy is produced.
:oxygen is not always necessary — since in the body hydrogen removal or dehydrogenation is most common.
:in the body carbohydrates serve as primary fuel and are oxidized to $Co_2 + H_2O$, with energy liberation.

pellagra: a disease due to a deficiency of the vitamin niacin, characterized by dermatitis, diarrhea, dementia, and eventually death if unremedied.

peristalsis: motions of the alimentary tract to move the food through the tract, characterized by alternate contraction and relaxation of muscle tissue from the esophagus to the intestines towards the anus.

peroxidation: formation of peroxide as a result of the action of oxygen on polyunsaturated fatty acids; vitamin E, a reducing agent, prevents lipid peroxidation in cells.

polyunsaturated fatty acids (PUFA): fatty acid containing two or more double bonds; linolenic and arachidonic acids.

recommended dietary (or daily) allowances (RDA): amounts of 15 vitamins and minerals plus protein and calories estimated to be needed for both sexes throughout the life cycle; allowances will maintain good nutrition in essentially all healthy persons in the United States under current living conditions; designed to afford a margin of safety above average physiological requirements to cover variations among individuals in the population; established by the Food and Nutrition Board of the National Academy of Sciences — National Research Council first in 1943 and revised several times as new research data become available.

seborrheic dermatitis: skin lesions characterized by greasy scaling, the condition may be a result of various factors such as oily skin, hormonal imbalance, emotional disturbance, and nutritional deficiency (as in riboflavin and pyriodoxine deficiencies).

somatic: pertaining to the body framework as distinguished from the viscera.

steatorrhea: presence of fat in stool, may be caused by defective fat absorption, lack of bile, or lack of lipase, a fat digestive enzyme.

transduce: to transfer genetically determined properties between microorganisms through the mediation of bacteriophage.

triglyceride: an ester of fatty acids and glycerol in which the glycerol molecule has three fatty acids attached to it; in over 98% of the fat found in foods.

United States recommended daily allowances (U.S. RDA): amounts of protein, 19 vitamins and minerals set by the Food and Drug Administration in 1973 as a revision of the MDR (minimum daily requirement) and utilizing the NAS/NRC (National Academy of Sciences/National Research Council) Recommended Dietary Allowances as a base; RDA table has been condensed to four categories; infants, children under four, adults and children over four years of age, and pregnant or lactating women, there is no consideration to sex or differentiation of age within these groups; generally the highest values in the NAS/NRC RDA table were selected for use within each U.S. RDA category; considering the margin of safety already built into the NAS/NRC's RDA, the U.S. RDA values are frequently higher than the needs of most people; individuals may only need 1/2 or 2/3 of the U.S. RDA for some nutrients, values determined primarily for use in labelling of foods.

viscera: organs of the digestive, respiratory, urogenital, and endocrine system as well as the spleen, the heart, and great vessels.

vitamin: organic compound occurring in minute amounts in foods; essential for numerous metabolic reactions; fat-soluble A, D, E and K; water-soluble ascorbic acid (C) and B complex.

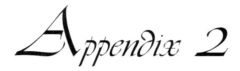

THE 7 DAY DIET*

A Computer-Analyzed Diet
For Older Americans

EVALUATION AND COMPARISON

This sample diet for older Americans was designed to provide for their special needs, aimed at health maintenance and energy levels for daily activities. The discussion which follows will concentrate on the statistics provided by a computer evaluation of the "major" nutrients, plus an additional consideration of zinc and fiber content.

*Prepared by
Mrs. Anne Bailey, M.S., Nutritionist

WATER

A 1968 DHEW report (Pub. No. HRA 74-1510), indicates that about 10% of Americans over 65 complain of chronic constipation. Generous intake of water and other liquids, plus adequate dietary fiber may contribute to the allevaition of this problem.

The computer-calculated water content of this tailored diet averaged 1785 grams daily, or about eight glasses, a reflection of the generous allowances of fruits and vegetables in various forms as well as milk and soups. Adding plain water, tea or coffee consumed, the total intake of liquids provides good support for the metabolic and excretory functions of a healthy older person.

CALORIES

The 1816 average daily caloric intake shown on the graph is essentially the 1974 RDA proposed for American females over 51 years of age. This diet could easily be modified to yield the 2400 calories recommended for males by simply increasing the amounts served, and with the addition of some of the suggested snacks or the inclusion of special desserts occasionally.

Since the 1800 calorie RDA is for the hypothetical "average" woman over 51, 65 inches tall and weighing 128 pounds, caloric adjustments are indicated for persons of varying heights and weights who wish to maintain their desirable body weight. For example, a larger, taller person would make adjustments, as suggested for males, such as larger portions and the addition of snacks.

Further, activities beyond or less than what most older persons experience change the daily calorie requirement. A 60 year old jogger obviously must have more calories if this is a routine part of his or her day. At the other extreme, the healthy, but delicate and lethargic individual would need to cut calories below 1800 to avoid excessive weight gain. Even severe climate, and variations in clothing, housing, and stress make enough difference to warrant consideration.

The smaller person must be especially careful not to reduce caloric intake to the point where particular nutrient deficiencies are created. A relationship between general health level and caloric intake was established in at least one study of women 40-70 years of age, with their health rated as poor when kcalorie consumption was between 1125 and 1475 (Guthrie, 1975). Nutrient density of food items chosen for this menu plan was used as a means for the determination of optimal amounts of these nutrients, rather than the gross addition of calories.

Dietary appraisal considers caloric intake and manipulation of these calories to achieve and maintain desirable weight by constant surveillance throughout life.

PROTEIN

The 1974 RDA for the "over 51" female is 46 grams of protein determined on the basis of .8gm/kg. However if her "average" weight is 128 pounds (approximately 58 kg) and calculation of one gram of protein per kg (original U.S. Food and Nutrition Board estimate) is made, the recommended amount of protein would total 58 grams per day.

In this menu plan, "she" averaged 86 grams of protein per day, or 86% above the 1974 RDA but just 48% above the more liberal recommendation of one gram of protein per kg of body weight. As recommended by Young (1976), this menu is closer to the gram per kilogram rule.

Comparing calories from proteins in this diet with the recommended 10-15%, (U.S. Public Health Service) we find 71 calories (26% above) in excess of the upper limit. The average caloric value of proteins in these menus is a balance which is generous, but acceptable.

The growing interest in vegetarianism and the fact that meat represents the costliest part of meals prompted an extra calculation. Protein values of all the meat items, when subtracted from the total, came to approximately 14 grams, bringing the total to 72 grams per day, still a generous amount. This was due to the fact that the remaining non meat proteins . . . dairy products, fish, eggs, nuts and legumes appear frequently throughout the week and provide the blend of essential amino acids needed for maintenance.

FATS

With an average daily total of 74 grams of fat, this diet

plan provides 666 calories or 37% of the total calories from fat sources, which is within the 40% top line suggested by many public health officials. Fat intake is important as a carrier of the fat-soluble vitamins as well as for its insulating, lubricating, cushioning and concentrated-energy source qualities.

Computer analysis revealed that 31%, slightly less than a third of these fats, were the saturated type. The essential fatty acids, linoleic and linolenic are well-supplied in almost equal amounts of 23 and 26 grams respectively. Calories from these two fatty acids add up to 342, which is close to the 2% (363 calories in this case) of total calories recommended for these essential fatty acids (Krause & Hunscher, 1972).

A final observation regarding this menu: it contains a minimum of "hidden fat" sources, such as fried foods, pastries and processed foods, and thus could provide a model for healthy choices in future meal plans.

CARBOHYDRATE

An examination of the printout information on carbohydrates supplied daily by this special menu revealed that the 220 gram average contributes 888 calories or 49% of the total caloric intake, which is just 1% short of the 50-58% carbohydrate range suggested by Dr. Jean Mayer. Most of these calories originate from the complex carbohydrates (whole grain breads and cereals) and from the fructose as supplied by fruits and fruit juices in the menu. These are preferred sources related to constipation and the achievement of good nutrient density, as well as a minimal of empty calorie carbohydrates typical with sucrose (cake toppings, pie etc.). The altered glucose tolerance explored in the monograph addresses the changes in carbohydrate metabolism that develop with advancing years. Suggested intake away from the refined sugars to the more complex carbohydrates (which are also significant sources of some regulatory nutrients) appears reasonable and appropriate.

CALCIUM

This special menu provides an average of 1388 mg per day for calcium, contributed mainly by the dairy products and green vegetables and is generously over the 800 mg RDA revision of 1974. Unfortunately, phosphorus was not included in the computer calculations, so the calcium/phosphrous ratio is not given, even though excess phosphate could tend to exaggerate bone loss (Jowsey, 1976).

For the elderly, it is still important to include generous amounts of calcium in the diet in order to minimize further damage to the skeleton, especially if there has been chronic deprivation of this mineral over a lifetime. (detailed discussion in monograph)

The absence of soft drinks and alcoholic beverages from this diet should improve calcium/phosphorus balance (1:1 or 2:1) and metabolism, because these drinks contain phosphorus (to supply the "fizz") and alcohol, which tends to reduce the absorption of calcium by one half (Jowsey, 1976).

IRON

This "older American" diet contains 14 mg of daily iron, on the average, a 40% addition to the Recommended Daily Allowance. The foods which contribute heavily to the amount of iron intake are such items as lentils, beef vegetable stew, whole grain bread, chicken livers, tuna, prunes and eggs. In the usual American diet, there are about six grams of iron per 1000 calories (Ho, 1971), so this plan provides well for this nutrient. Intestinal absorption of iron is generally poor (about 10% of intake) and losses occur through the urine, feces and sweat glands in the amount of approximately a gram per day.

Most mineral elements are well distributed in foods, but iron and calcium are the exceptions. California passed a bill in January of 1972 which requires iron enrichment of flour, bread, cereal and products containing 25% or more of any grain. The inclusion of these products in the diet also helps meet iron requirements for Californian retirees. The nutritional anemias are discussed in detail in the monograph.

ZINC

Zinc is the most recent (1974) trace mineral for which an RDA has been established ... 25 mg daily. In his interesting discussion of trace minerals Labuza (1975) concludes: "Zinc given orally is a useful therapeutic agent in peripheral vascular disease, even with gangrene and also has favorable effects on ischemic hearts and brains."

Marginal zinc intakes are attributed to increased consumption of sugars, fats and refined grains. The zinc content of foods can be extremely variable. For example, 100 gram portions of oysters, when tested, yielded numbers from 15.9 to 207.0 mg of zinc. Data on the zinc content of foods are incomplete, but major sources are those of animal origin such as eggs, meat, dairy products, poultry and fish. Bran and wheat germ, peanuts and mature dry legumes are also good sources.

The estimated zinc content of this diet was calculated at an average of 14 mg. per day, 93% of the present Recommended Daily Allowance.

THE VITAMINS
Vitamin A

A glance at the graph reveals generous intakes of vitamin A, thiamin, riboflavin, niacin and ascorbic acid, the five vitamins included in this analysis.

Because the fat-soluble vitamin A can be stored in the liver, individuals can "coast" on this reserve supply through days or even months of inadequate intake. Following this menu would provide almost twice the Recommended Daily Allowance of 4000 International Units and allow for this kind of cushioning. Foods making substantial contributions of vitamin A are liver and margarine, plus fruits and vegetables such as watermelon, plums, spinach and carrots.

Using the 1972 ten-state survey figure for females of 196 International Inits per 100 kcalories, the usual total for vitamin A from foods would be 3525, well below what is provided in this special diet.

Toxicity from overconsumption of vitamin A or any of the vitamins is possible. This may be especially true for those individuals taking self-prescribed, nutritional supplements. It is one thing to consume a diet rich in essential nutrients and quite another matter when serious imbalances are created in the "pill-poppers" (with resulting side effects) by their ignorance, gullibility or cavalier attitude.

THE VITAMIN B COMPLEX

Of the three B vitamins analyzed, the high level of riboflavin (174% of the RDA) is attributed to the generous inclusion of dairy products in this diet. Although just three of the complex group are represented here, if thiamin and riboflavin are provided for adequately in a balanced diet, the rest of the B vitamins will also be adequate.

Physiological inefficiency in utilizing these vitamins plus the possible adverse effects (increased excretion of vitamins) of certain therapeutic drugs may account for increased need for thiamin and other vitamins.

Further, the elderly person who is more active than usual may especially benefit from the high level of B vitamins found in this diet, since thiamin and niacin, both coenzymes in many enzymatic reactions, are required for synthesis and energy production.

ASCORBIC ACID

The exact 'geriatric' requirement for ascorbic acid has not been ascertained; its total participation in bodily metabolic processes is still to be defined. Deficiency states in the aged could be critical since the body cannot synthesize vitamin C. There are frequent reports of extremely low ascorbic acid intake among the elderly (see monograph). Vitamin C has been identified as involved in many reactions, but some of the most important are:

collagen synthesis

deposition and withdrawal of calcium in bones and teeth

synthesis of thyroxin, regulation of metabolic rate

production of adrenal hormones

The 119 mg average of ascorbic acid obtained from foods on this menu is a high value as compared with the 45 mg of the 1974 RDA and is derived from such foods as strawberries, grapefruit, oranges and broccoli.

Water soluble vitamins are not stored and excess is

excreted in the urine. Only scattered studies of vitamin C toxicity have been reported, so that the value herein calculated does not appear excessive.

DIETARY FIBER

At this time, the recommended daily allowance (RDA) for fiber has not been established for any age group, but interest in this "nutrient" continues to mount as bits and pieces of evidence are put together to identify potential benefits from its use.

In gerontology, there is concern with gastro-intestinal health problems. Any preventive and/or therapeutic value that may result from dietary fiber has been (and is) studied.

Caution may be necessary, however, by persons with gastro-intestinal problems. One should also be aware of the physiological effects. It is possible that large amounts of fiber-containing foods may affect serum levels of ionized calcium, iron and cholesterol (Persson et al., 1976).

At least 100 mg (6 grams) of fiber per kg of body weight has been suggested as a standard for aiding elimination (Guthrie, 1975). Recently, 10 to 12 grams of crude fiber intake was advised (Labuza, 1977).

Although fiber content of this diet was not analyzed by a computer program, the inclusion of items such as whole grain breads, brown rice, oatmeal, bran muffins, salads and other fruits and vegetables will provide the bulk and moisture-absorbing capacity needed for "regularity." Further there are few refined, processed or "convenience" foods in this selection, thus increasing the proportion of unrefined, high-residue foods in their natural state.

OLDER AMERICAN TAILORED DIET – FEMALE   PERSONAL INFO CODE: 55, 7 DAYS

NUTRIENT LEVELS COMPARED TO RECOMMENDED DIETARY ALLOWANCES (1974 RDA)

	WT GM	H2O GM	CAL	PRTN GM	FAT GM	FATTY ACIDS – SAID OLEIC		GM LINO	CHO GM	CA MG	FE MG	VIT A IU	THIA MG	RFLVN MG	NICN MG	ASC MG
TOTALS	15474	12496	12709	599	516	159	180	81	1539	9713	98.0	81411	9.91	21.07	112.8	836
DAILY AVRGE	2211	1785	1816	86	74	23	26	12	220	1388	14.0	11630	1.42	3.01	16.1	119
RECOMMENDED			1800	46						800	10.0	4000	1.00	1.10	12.0	45
DIFFERENCE			16	40						588	4.0	7630	0.42	1.91	4.1	74
PERCENT DIFFERENCE			1	86						73	40	191	42	174	34	166

```
100 +
    +
 80 +
    +
 60 +
    +
 40 +
    +
 20 +
ACCEPTABLE   +
    +
RECOMMENDED  0 +
    +
-20 +
ACCEPTABLE   +
-40 +
    +
-60 +
    +
-80 +
    +
-100 +
```

This chart is a graphic representation of computer calculation results when the special 7-day diet was analyzed. Information on these pages details major nutrient contributions of different food items on the menu, with food code numbers taken from the U.S. Home and Garden Bulletin number 72. **Nutritive Value of Foods,** U.S. Government Printing Office, Washington, D.C., 1971.

GUIDELINES AND MEAL PATTERNS
FOR OLDER PERSONS

Try, each day, for *at least:*

*** 1 serving each meal of whole grain cereal, bread or macaroni product

*** 2 glasses of milk or its equivalent, such as yogurt, eggnog, milk shake, puddings, custard, ice cream, cheese or soups.

*** 2 servings of meat or meat substitutes of high quality protein such as beef, pork, lamb, fish, eggs, poultry, peas, beans, legumes, nuts and seeds.

*** 2 servings of fruit, including at least one which is rich in vitamin C.

*** 2 servings of vegetables, one of which should be a leafy, dark green type.

*** 8 glasses of liquids, including water. Tea, coffee, milk, consomme, soups, fruit juices and watery fruits and vegetables can all contribute to this total.

Note: An average serving of bread is one slice.
An average serving of cereal is 1/2 to 3/4 cup.
An average serving of fruits or vegetables is at least 1/2 cup.
An average serving of cooked meat is three ounces.

Meal patterns can be used as check lists for nutritional adequacy. Here are some examples:

BREAKFAST	LUNCH
Fruit	Main dish from meat group
Egg or cereal or both	Vegetable
Toast or hotbread and butter	Bread and butter
Milk	Fruit

DINNER

Main dish from meat group	Potato
Other vegetable	Bread or hotbread w/butter
Milk	Dessert

Snacks could make healthy additions to daily food intake and if modified and selected according to individual caloric and other needs. If preferred, total food intake can be divided into five or six small meals. This may prove inconvenient, but does provide advantages such as easier digestion, less chance of over-eating or, conversely, of nutritional deprivation over a period of several hours.

References: Menu for Older Persons

Adams, C.F. *Nutritive value of American foods in common units.* Agriculture Handbook No. 456. Washington, D.C.: U.S. Department of Agriculture, Government Printing Office, 1975.

Albanese, A.A. Nutrition and health of the elderly. *Nutrition News.* Rosemont, IL.: National Dairy Council, 1976, *39*(2) 5,8.

Almy, T.P. The role of fiber in the diet. In M. Winick, *Nutrition and Aging,* New York: John Wiley and Sons, 1976, 155-169.

Burton, B.T. *Human nutrition* (3rd edition) New York: McGraw-Hill Book Company (published for H.J. Heinz Company), 1976.

Guthrie, H.A. *Introductory nutrition.* St. Louis: The C.V. Mosby Company, 1975, 25.

Haeflein, J.A. and Rasmussen, A.I. Zinc content of selected foods. *Journal of the American Dietetic Association,* 1977, *70*(6), 610-615.

Ho, G.P. What is your iron score. *Nutrition Highlights,* USDA Extension, 1971, May.

Jowsey, J.J. Prevention and treatment of osteoporosis. In M. Winick (Ed.), *Nutrition and aging,* New York: John Wiley and Sons, 1976, 131-144.

Krause, M.V. and Hunscher, M.A. *Food, nutrition and diet therapy,* (5th edition) Philadelphia: W.D. Saunders Company, 1972, 64.

Labuza, T.P. *Food and your well being.* Los Angeles: West Publishing Company, 1977, 50.

Labuza, T.P. *The nutrition crisis.* Los Angeles: West Publishing Company, 1975, 355-373.

Mayer, J. *A diet for living.* New York: David McKay Company, Inc. 1975.

Murphy, E.W., Willis, B.W. and Watt, B.K. Provisional tables on the zinc content of foods. *Journal of the American Dietetic Association,* 1975, *66*(4) 345-355.

National Research Council, Food and Nutrition Board, *Recommended dietary allowances,* 8th revised edition, Washington, D.C.: National Academy of Sciences, 1974.

Nutrition of the elderly. *Dairy Council Digest.* Rosemont, Il.: National Dairy Council, 1977, *48* (1), 1-5.

Nutritive value of foods, Home and garden bulletin No. 72, Washington, D.C.: U.S. Department of Agriculture. U.S. Government Printing Office, 1971.

Persson, I., Raby, K., Fonss-Bech, P. and Jensen, E. Effect of prolonged administration on serum levels of cholesterol, ionized calcium and iron in the elderly. *American Geriatric Society, 24,* 334.

Peterkin, B., Nichols, J. and Cromwell, C. *Nutrition labeling, tools for its use.* Agriculture Information Bulletin No. 382, Washington, D.C.: Consumer and Food Economics Institute, Agricultural Research Service, U.S. Department of Agriculture, Superintendent of Documents, U.S. Government Printing Office, 1975.

Robertson, L., Flinders, C. and Godfry, B. *Laurel's Kitchen.* Berkeley, CA.: Nilgiri Press, 1976, 454-456.

Watt, B.C. and Merrill, A.L. *Composition of foods,* Agriculture Handbook No. 8, Washington, D.C.: USDA Agricultural Research Service, U.S. Government Printing Office, 1963.

Whitney, E. and Hamilton, M. *Understanding Nutrition,* Los Angeles: West Publishing Company, 1977.

Young, V.R. Protein metabolism and needs in elderly people. In M. Rockstein and M.L. Sussman (eds.), *Nutrition, longevity and aging.* New York: Academic Press, 1976, 67-102.

SEVEN DAYS OF GOOD EATING
TAILOR-MADE MEAL PLANS FOR OLDER PERSONS

MONDAY

Breakfast
  grape juice — 4 oz.
  apple pancakes — 4 med.
  sausage — 2 links

Lunch
  lentil soup — 1 cup
  pumpernickel toast with
    margarine — 1 slice
  skim milk — 8 oz.
  fresh pear — medium

Dinner
  tuna/noodle/peas casserole — 1 cup
  broccoli with mock hollandaise sauce — ¾ cup
  cabbage/carrot coleslaw — 1/3 cup
  fresh or canned pineapple slice — 1
  cottage cheese — 2/3 cup
  herb tea with lemon

Snack suggestions
  orange juice malt
  cheese-spread stuffed celery

TUESDAY

Breakfast
  sliced banana in pineapple
    juice — ½ banana,
    4 oz. juice
  cooked Wheatena — ½ cup,
    with raisins/brown
    sugar, milk
  2 slices broiled canadian
    bacon
  eggnog — 1 cup

Lunch
  minestrone — 1 cup
  rye wafers/margarine
  peanut butter-stuffed celery
    sticks
  walnut-topped prunes — 4
  buttermilk — 8 oz.

Dinner
  beef/vegetable stew — 1 cup
  tossed salad with yogurt dressing — 1 cup
  V-8 tomato juice cocktail — 4 oz.
  tea or coffee

Snack suggestions
  wheat thins with cheddar cheese
  low-fat fruit yogurt

WEDNESDAY

Breakfast
  sliced fresh orange — 1 med.
  creamed chipped beef and
    hard-cooked egg on
    wheat toast
  skim milk — 8 oz.
  Sanka — 1 cup

Lunch
  celery/apple/date/walnut salad —
    ¾ cup
  rye wafers with margarine
  skim milk — 8 oz.

Dinner
  pork chop with rice — 1 cup
  glazed carrots with orange — ½ cup
  fresh or canned plums — 3
  tea or coffee

Snack suggestions
  strawberry ice milk
  dehydrated fruit roll

THURSDAY

Breakfast
  cranberry juice cocktail —
    4 oz.
  whole wheat french
    toast — 2 slices
  plain yogurt — 8 oz.

Lunch
  cheese pizza — 1 med. wedge
  3 bean salad — 1 cup
  skim milk — 1 cup

Dinner
  6-minute crispy chicken livers — 3 oz.
  brown rice — 2/3 cup
  spinach with mushrooms — ½ cup
  fresh blueberries — ¾ cup
    (or other fruit in season)
  herb tea with lemon

Snack suggestions
  toasted bagel with cheese spread
  hiker's mix (snipped dried fruits, nuts, cereal bits, chocolate bits,
    raisins, etc.)

FRIDAY

Breakfast
stewed prunes — 4 large
cooked oatmeal with sliced
  banana, brown sugar —
  ½ cup
jack cheese — 1 slice
cocoa, made with skim
  milk — 8 oz.

Lunch
tuna-relish spread on whole
  wheat bun
carrot sticks
skim milk — 8 oz.

Dinner
turkey potroast dinner — 1 cup
blender spinach soup — 2/3 cup
melon slice or canned peaches
Sanka or coffee

Snack suggestions
banana, yogurt, apricot nectar blend
mixed nuts

SATURDAY

Breakfast
fresh strawberries — 2/3 cup
wheat flakes with dates —
  ½ cup
slice cheddar cheese
skim milk — 8 oz.

Lunch
cottage cheese and fresh fruit
  salad
bran muffin
banana chips
herb tea

Dinner
broiled fish filet — 3 oz.
spanish rice — ½ cup
zucchini with parmesan cheese — 2/3 cup
in-season melon slice

Snack suggestions
liverwurst on cracker
grapefruit/orange juice blend

SUNDAY

Breakfast
   pink grapefruit — ½
   poached egg on whole wheat
      toast, topped with cheese
   plain yogurt
   hot tea

Lunch
   fish chowder made with 2% milk
      — 1 cup
   peanut/carrot/pickle salad —
      ½ cup
   corn muffin with margarine
   apple juice — 4 oz.

Dinner
   easy chili — 1 cup
   molded lime jello, fruit, cottage cheese salad
   baked custard — 2/3 cup
   coffee or tea

Snack suggestions
   dried apricots with almonds
   beef jerky

ACKNOWLEDGMENT:

Without the gracious assistance of Frank R. Little, M.S., Business Data Processing Department of Santa Monica College (California), the computerized nutrient evaluation of the Diet for Older Americans would not have been possible. Our special thanks and appreciation to Frank Little for his valuable contribution.

EXPLANATION OF SYMBOLS

Lack of space does not permit the use of complete words for identifying nutrients which were computer-analyzed. The two lists which appear below may be helpful to the reader not familiar with these column headings.

CONTRACTION   TERM

AMT UNITS . . . . amount in units
WT GM . . . . weight in grams
H20 GM . . . . .water, in grams
CAL . . . . .kilocalories
PRTN GM . . . . .protein, in grams
FAT GM . . . . grams of fat
FATTY ACIDS . . GM . . . . fatty acids, in grams
SATD   . . . . saturated
OLEIC . . . . oleic acid (an essential fatty acid)
LINO . . . . linoleic acid (an essential fatty acid)
CHO GM . . . . .carbohydrate, in grams
CA MG . . . . calcium, in milligrams
FE MG . . . . iron, in milligrams
VIT A IU . . . . vitamin A, international units
THIA MG . . . . thiamin, in milligrams
RELVN MG . . . . riboflavin, in milligrams
NICN MG . . . . niacin, in milligrams
ASC MG . . . . .ascorbic acid, in milligrams

REFERENCES CITED

Abramsky, O. Common and uncommon neurological manifestations as presenting symptoms of vitamin B_{12} deficiency. *Journal of the American Geriatric Society,* 1972, *20*(2), 93-96.

Adler, W. H. Aging and the immune function. *Biological Science,* 1975, 25(10), 652-657.

Agate, J. Diseases of deprivation. *Proceedings of the Royal Society of Medicine,* 1968, *61*(9), 919-22.

Agate, J. The Natural history of disease in later life. In I. Rossman (Ed.), *Clinical Geriatrics.* Philadelphia: J. B. Lippincott Co., 1971, 115-120.

Albanese, A. A. General nutrition of the aging patient with some observations on specific metabolic needs. In J. T. Freeman (Ed.), *Clinical Principals and Drugs in the Aging.* Springfield, Ill.: Thomas, 1963, 173-218.

Albanese, A. A. Nutritional aspects of bone loss. *Food and Nutrition News,* 1975, *47*(2), 1-4.

Albright, F., Smith, P. H. and Richardson, A. M. Postmenopausal osteoporosis: Its clinical features. *Journal of the American Medical Association,* 1941, *116*(22), 2465.

Albrink, M. J., Davidson, P. C. and Newman, T. Lipid-lowering effect of a very high carbohydrate high-fiber diet. Annual meeting of the American Diabetes Association, San Francisco, 1976.

Albrink, M. J., Meigs, J. W., and Granoff, M. A. Weight gains and serum triglycerides in normal men. *New England Journal of Medicine,* 1962, *266,* 484.

Almy, T. P. The role of fiber in the diet. In M. Winick (Ed.), *Nutrition and Aging.* New York: John Wiley & Sons, 1976, 155-170.

Anderson, W. F. Unanswered questions in the nutrition of elderly people. *Proceedings of the Nutrition Society* (England), 1968, *27*(2), 185-7.

Andres, R., Pozefsky, T., Swerdloff, R. S. and Tobin, J. D. Effect of aging on carbohydrate metabolism. In R. A.

Camerini-Davalos and H. S. Cole (Eds.), *Early Diabetes.* New York: Academic Press, 1970, 349-355.

Andres, R. and Tobin, J. Aging and the disposition glucose. In Cristofalo *et al.* (Eds.), *Explorations in Aging.* New York: Plenum Publishing Co., 1975, 239.

Andrews, J. and Brook, M. Leucocyte-vitamin C content and clinical signs in the elderly. *The Lancet,* 1966, *1*(7451), 1350-1.

Arey, L. B., Tremain, M. J. and Monzingo, F. L. The numerical and topographical relation of taste buds to human circumvallate papillae throughout the life span. *Anatomical Record*, 1935, *64,* 9-25.

Baker, A. Z. Some observations on the nutritional intake of patients in long-stay geriatric units. *Gerontologia Clinica,* 1962, *4,* 100-7.

Balsley, M., Brink, M. F. and Speckmann, E. W. Nutrition in disease and stress. *Geriatrics,* 1971, *26*(3), 87-93.

Barndt, R. Jr., Blankenhorn, D. H., Crawford, D. W., Brooks, S. H. Regression and Progression of Early Femoral Atherosclerosis in treated hyperlipoproteinemic patients. *Annals of Internal Medicine,* 1977, *86*:139-146.

Batata, M., Spray, G. H., Bolton, F. G., Higgins, G. and Wollner, L. Blood and bone marrow changes in elderly patients with special reference to folic acid, vitamin B$_{12}$, iron, and ascorbic acid. *British Medical Journal,* 1967, *2,* 667.

Beaudoin, R., Van Itallie, T. B. and Mayer, J. Carbohydrate metabolism in "active" and "static" human obesity. *American Journal of Clinical Nutrition,* 1953, *1*(2), 91.

Bender, A. E. Nutrition of the elderly. *Royal Society of Health Journal (England),* 1971a, *91*(3), 115-21.

Bender, A. E., Damji, K B. In J. Yudkin, J. Edelman and L. Hough (Eds.) *Sugar, Chemical Biological and Nutritional Aspects of Sucrose.* London: Butterworths, 1971b.

Bergami, G. The problem of excess weight in the elderly. *Panminerva Medica (Torino),* 1965, *7,* 321-3.

Berman, P. M. and Kirsner, J. B. The aging gut: Diseases of the esophagus, small intestine, and appendix. *Geriatrics,* 1972a, *27*(3), 84-90.

Berman, P. M. and Kirsner, J. B. The aging gut: Diseases of the colon, pancreas, liver, and gallbladder. Functional bowel disease and iatrogenic disease. *Geriatrics,* 1972b, *27*(4), 117-24.

Bermond, P. Letter: Clinical symptoms of malnutrition and plasma ascorbic acide levels. *American Journal of Clinical Nutrition,* 1976, *29*(5), 493.

Bieri, J. G. Vitamin E. In *Present Knowledge in Nutrition,* 1976, pp. 98-110 (p. 104, 105).

Bierman, E. L. Fat metabolism, atherosclerosis and aging in man: A review. *Mechanisms of Aging and Development,* 1973, *2*, 315.

Bierman, E. L. Obesity, carbohydrate and lipid interactions in the elderly. In M. Winick (Ed.), *Nutrition and Aging.* New York: John Wiley & Sons, 1976.

Bigwood, E. J. Senescence and nutrition. An important sociological and economic problem of actuality to nutritionists. *Nutritio et Dieta (Switzerland),* 1966, *8*, 226-34.

Bigwood, E. J. What is a dietetic food? *Bibliotheca Nutritio et Dieta,* 1973, *18*, 165-70.

Bjorntorp, P., Gahlen, M., Grimby, G., Gustafson, A., Holm, J., Renstrom, P. and Schernsten, T. Carbohydrate and lipid metabolism in middle-aged, physically well-trained men. *Metabolism-Clinical and Experimental,* 1972, *21*(11), 1037-1044.

Blackburn, G. L., Flatt, J. P., Clowes, G. A. A., Jr., *et al.* Protein in sparing therapy during periods of starvation with sepsis or trauma. *Annals of Surgery,* 1973, *177*, 588-594.

Blackman, A. H., Lambert, D. L., Thayer, W.R., *et al.* Computed normal values for peak acide output based on age, sex, and body weight. *American Journal of Digestive Diseases,* 1970, *15*, 783.

Bogert, L. J., Briggs, G. M. and Calloway, D. H. *Nutrition and Physical Fitness.* Philadelphia: Saunders, 1973.

Briggs, G. Quotes from newspaper report of comments of the 4th Annual Nutrition Conference of Dairy Council of California, *Los Angeles Times,* April 4, 1974.

Briggs, G. M. Sugar, nutrition and disease, addendum to testimony at hearing before California Senate Subcommittee on Agriculture, Food, Nutrition. San Francisco, 1974.

Brin, M. Biochemical methods and findings in USA surveys. In A. N. Exton-Smith, and D. L. Scott (Eds.), *Vitamins in the Elderly*. Bristol: John Wright & Sons, Ltd., 1968.

Brin, M., Dibble, M. V., Peel, A., McMullen, E., Bourquin, A., and Chen, N. Some preliminary findings on the nutritional status of the aged in Onondaga County, New York, *American Journal of Clinical Nutrition,* 1965, *17*(4), 240-58.

Brin, M., Schwartzberg, S. H., and Arthur-Davis, D. A vitamin evaluation program as applied to 10 elderly residents in a community home for the aged. *Journal of the American Geriatrics Society,* 1964, *12,* 493-9.

Brink, M. F., Speckman, E. W. and Balsley, M. Current concepts in geriatric nutrition. *Geriatrics,* 1968, *23*(3), 113-20.

British Dept. of Health and Social Security. Recommended intakes of nutrients for the United Kingdom. London: Her Majesty's Stationery Office, 1972.

British Medical Journal, Old Age, nutrition, and mental confusion. 1969, *3*(5671), 608.

Brocklehurst, J. C. (Ed.) *Textbook of Geriatric Medicine and Gerontology.* London: Churchill Livingstone, 1973.

Bronte-Stewart, B., Roberts, B., Wells, V. W. Serum cholesterol in vitamin C deficiency in man. *British Journal of Nutrition,* 1963, *17*(1), 61-8.

Brook, M., Brimshaw, J. J. Vitamin C concentration of plasma and leucocytes relating to smoking habit, age and sex of humans. *American Journal of Clinical Nutrition,* 1968, *21*(11), 1254-8.

Brooks, A. L., Mead, D. K. and Peters, R. F. Effects of aging on the frequency of metaphase chromosome aberrations in the liver of the Chinese hamster. *Journal of Gerontology,* 1973, *28*(4), 452-454.

Brozek, J. Physique and nutritional status of adult men. *Human Biology,* 1956, *28-29,* 124-40.

Bullamore, J. R., Gallagher, J. C., Wilkinson, R., Nordin, B. E. C., and Marshall, D. H. Effect of age on calcium absorption. *The Lancet,* 1970, *2*(7672), 535-537.

Burkitt, D. P.   Epidemiology of cancer of colon and rectum. *Cancer* 1971, *28*,3.

Burkitt, D. P., Walker, A. R. P., and Painter, N. S.   Effect of dietary fibre on stools and transit times and its role in the causation of disease. *The Lancet,* 1972, *2*, 1408.

Burkitt, D. P.   Some disease characteristics of modern western civilization. *British Medical Journal, 1973, 1,* 274.

Burnett, M.   *Intrinsic Mutagensis. A Genetic Approach to Aging.* New York: Wiley & Sons, 1974, 244.

Burr, M. L., Hurley, R. J. and Sweetman, P. M.   Vitamin supplementation of old people with low blood levels. *Gerontologic Clinica* (Basel), 1975, *17*(4), 236-243.

Burton, B. T.   Human nutrition and aging. In F. C. Jeffers (Ed.), *Duke University Council on Gerontology. Proceedings of Seminars, 1961-1965.* Durham: Duke University Regional Center for Study of Aging, 1965, 24-39.

Burton, B. T.   Fluid, electrolyte, and acid base balance. *Human Nutrition.* New York: McGraw-Hill, 1976, 15-19.

Butler, R.   *Why Survive? Being Old in America.* San Francisco: Harper & Row, 1975.

Byrd, E. and Gertman, S.   Taste sensitivity in aging persons. *Geriatrics,* 1959, *14,* 381.

Call, D. L. and Sanchez, A. M.   Trends in fat diasppearance in the United States. *Journal of Nutrition,* 1967, *93*(2), 1-28.

Callender, S. T.   Iron absorption from food. *Gerontologica Clinics,* 1971, *13*, 44-51.

Cameron, E. and Pauling, L.   Ascorbic acide and the glycosaminoglycans and orthomolecular approach to cancer and other diseases. *Oncology,* 1973, *27,* 181-92.

Carlson, M. P. and Bottiger, E.   Ischaemic heart disease in relation to fasting values of plasma triglycerides and cholesterol. *The Lancet,* 1972, *1,* 865.

Carrel, A. and Ebeling, A. H.   Age and multiplication of fibroglasts. *Journal of Experimental Medicine,* 1921, *34*(6) 599-623.

Carruthers, M.   *The Western Way of Death.* London: Davis-Paynter, Ltd., 1974.

Chazan, J. A. and Mistilis, S. P. The pathophysiology of scurvy. *American Journal of Medicine,* 1963, *34*(3), 350-8.

Cheraskin, E., Ringsdorf, W. M., Jr., Michael, C. W., *et al.* Daily vitamin C consumption and reported respiratory findings. *International Journal of Vitamin Nutrition and Research,* 1973, *43,* 42-55.

Cheraskin, E., Ringsdorf, W. M., Jr., Setyaadmadja, A. T. and Barrett, E. A. Thiamin-carbohydrate consumption and cardiovascular complaints. *Internationale Zeitschrift Fuer Vitaminforschune* (Switzerland), 1967, *37,* 449-55.

Chernish, S. M., Helmer, O. M., Fouts, P. J. and Kohlstaedt, K. G. The effect of the intrinsic factor on absorption of vitamin B_{12} in older people. *American Journal of Clinical Nutrition,* 1957, *5,* 651-8.

Cheung, A. Personal communication with Dr. A. Cheung of the University of Southern California, School of Pharmacy, 1977.

Chope, H. D. Relation of nutrition to health in aging persons: A 4-year follow-up of a study of San Mateo County. *California Medicine,* 1954, *81*(5), 335-8.

Clayson, D. B. Nutrition and experimental carcinogenesis: A review. Paper presented at the Conference on "Nutrition in the Causation of Cancer," Key Biscayne, Florida, 1975.

Clemens, J. A., Amenoamori, Y., Jenkins, T. and Meites, J. Effects of hypothalamic stimulation, hormones and drugs on ovarian function in old female rats. *Society of experimental Biological Medicine,* 1969, *132,* 561.

Clements, F. W. Nutrition 7: Vitamin and mineral supplementation. *Medical Journal of Australia,* 1975, *1*(19), 595-9.

Clifford, G. Hematological problems in the elderly. In I. Rossman (Ed.), *Clinical Geriatrics.* Philadelphia: J. B. Lippincott Co., 1971, 253-266.

Coffee, G. and Wilson, C. W. M. Ascorbic acid deficiency and aspirin induced Haematemesis. *British Medical Journal,* 1975, *1,* 208.

Cohen, S. Geriatric Drug Abuse. In a Seminar "The Process and Treatment of Aging." *Drug Abuse and Alcoholism*

Newsletter. Vista Hill Foundation, 1975, IV(2).

Cohn, C. Meal eating, nibbling, and body metabolism. *Journal of the American Dietetic Association,* 1961, *38,* 433.

Cohn, C. Feeding patterns and some aspects of cholesterol metabolism. *Federation Proceedings,* 1964, *23*(1-2), 76-81.

Comfort, A. *Ageing: The Biology of Senescence.* New York: Holt, Rinehart and Winston, 1964.

Connell, A. M., Hilbon, C., Irvine, G., *et al.* Variations in bowel habit in two population samples. *British Medical Journal,* 1965, 2, 1095.

Consumer Reports. Vitamin E: What's behind all those claims for it? 1973, *38*(1), 60-64.

Cooper, R. M., Bilash, I. and Zubek, J. P. The effect of age on taste sensitivity. *Journal of Gerontology,* 1959, *14,*56-58.

Copeland, C. L. Dietary fibre: Search for the facts. *British Medical Journal,* 1975, *4,* 404.

Corless, D. Diet in the elderly. *British Medical Journal,* 1973, *4*(885), 158-60.

Corless, D., Boucher, B. J., Cohen, R. D., Beer, M. and Gupta, S. P. Vitamin D status in long-stay geriatric patients. *The Lancet,* 1975, *1*(7922), 1404-6.

Cosper, B. A. Personal and social factors related to food choices and eating behavior of selected young to middle-aged adults. *Dissertation Abstracts International,* 1973, *33*(12-B), 5937.

Crowley, G. and Curtis, H. J. The development of somatic mutations in mice with age. *Procedures of the National Academy of Science, United States of America,* 1963, *49,* 626-628.

Cummings, J. H., *et al.* Laxative-induced diarrhea: A continuing clinical problem. *British Medical Journal,* 1974, *1,* 537-541.

Curtis, H. J. The nature of the aging process. In E. Bittar and N. Bittar (Eds.), *The Biological Basis of Medicine.* London: Academic Press, Inc., 1968.

Cutler, C. W., Jr. Clinical patterns of peptic ulcer after 60. *Surgery, Gynecology and Obstetrics,* 1958, *107,* 23.

Cutler, R. G. Redundancy of information content in the genome of mammalian species as a protective mechanism determining aging rats. *Mechanisms of Aging and Human Development,* 1974, *2,* 381-408.

Dairy Council Digest. Nutrition, diet and cancer, 1975, *46*(5).

Dalderup, L. M., Van Dam, B. E., Schiedt, K., Keller, G. H. M. and Shouten, F. Intake of vitamins and some other nutrients in aged people, adults and children. *International Journal of Vitamin and Nutrition Research,* 1970, *40,* 633-643.

Dall, J. L. C. and Gardner, H. S. Dietary intake of potassium by geriatric patients. *Gerontologia Clinica (Basel),* 1971, *13*(3), 119-24.

Davies, D. Advances toward understanding diabetes mellitus. *Geriatrics,* 1975, *30*(1), 79-83.

Davis, M. E., Strandford, N. M. and Lanzl, L. H. Estrogens and the aging process. *Journal of the American Medical Association,* 1966, *196,* 219.

Davis, R. A., Gershoff, S. M. and Gamble, D. F. Review of study of vitamin and mineral nutrition in the United States, 1950-68. *Journal of Nutrition Education,* 1969, *1*(2), 41-57.

Davison, W. The hazards of drug treatment on old age. In J. C. Brocklehurst (Ed.), *Textbook of Geriatric Medicine and Gerontology.* London: Churchill Livingstone, 1973, 632-648.

Dent, C. E. and Watson, L. Osteoporosis. *Post Graduate Medical Journal,* 1966, *42.* (Supplement) 581.

Dibble, M. V., Brin, M., Thiele, V. F., Peel, A., Chen, N. and McMullen, E. Evaluation of the nutritional status of elderly subjects, with a comparison between fall and spring. *Journal of the American Geriatrics Society,* 1967, *15*(11), 1031-61.

Dilman, V. M. Age-associated elevation of hypothalamic threshold to feedback control and its role in development, aging and disease. *The Lancet,* 1971, *I,* 1211-1219.

DiLuzio, N. R. Antioxidants, lipid peroxidation and chemical-induced liver injury. *Federation Proceedings,* 1973, *32*(8), 1875-1881.

Duckworth, W. C. and Kitabachi, A. E. Direct measurement of plasma pro-insulin in normal and diabetic subjects. *American Journal of Medicine,* 1972, *53,* 418-427.

Durnin, J. V. G. A. Energy – requirements, intake and balance. *Proceedings of the Nutrition Society,* 1968, *27*(2), 188-91.

Eastwood, M. A. The role of vegetable dietary fibre in human nutrition. *Medical Hypotheses,* 1975, *1*(46), 46-53.

Eastwood, M. A. Fibre and enterohepatic circulation. *Nutrition Review,* 1977, *35*(3), 42-44.

Eckhardt, R. D. and Davidson, C. S. The oral and parenteral phenylalanine requirements for nitrogen equilibrium in man. *Journal of Clinical Investigation,* 1948, *27*(2) 165-70.

Elek, S. R. Stress Physiology Bulletin of Beverly Hills District, Los Angeles County Medical Association, 1970.

Elwood, T. W. Nutritional concerns of the elderly. *Journal of Nutrition Education,* 1975, *7*(2), 50-2.

Enstrom, J. E. Cancer mortality among Mormons. *Cancer,* 1975, *36,* 825.

Ericsson, P. The effect of iron supplementation on the physical work capacity of the elderly. *Acta Medica Scandinavica,* 1970, *188,* 361-74.

Exton-Smith, A. N. Health and nutrition of the elderly. *Royal Scoiety for the Promotion of Health Journal (London),* 1968a, *88*(4), 205-8.

Exton-Smith, A. N. The problem of subclinical malnutrition in the elderly. In A. N. Exton-Smith, and D. L. Scott (Eds.), *Vitamins in the Elderly.* Briston: Wright and Sons, Ltd., 1968b, 12-18.

Exton-Smith, A. N. Physiological aspects of aging: Relationship to nutrition. *American Journal of Clinical Nutrition,* 1972, *25*(8), 853-9.

Exton-Smith, A. N. Nutritional deficiencies in the elderly. In A. N. Howard and I. McLean (Eds.), *Nutritional Deficiencies in Modern Society.* London: Baird Newman, 1973.

Exton-Smith, A. N. and Stanton, B. R. *Report of an investigation in the dietary of elderly women living alone.* London: King Edward's Hospital Fund, 1965.

Exton-Smith, A. N. and Windsor, A. C. M. Principles of drug treatment in the aged. In I. Rossman (Ed.), *Clinical Geriatrics.* Philadelphia: J. B. Lippincott Co., 1971, 369-389.

Fabry, P., Fodor, J., Hejl, Z., Braun, T. and Zvolankova, K. The frequency of meals: Its relationship to overweight, hypercholesterolemia, and decreased glucose-tolerance. *The Lancet,* 1964, *2*(7360), 614-5.

Fabry, P., Fodor, J., Hejl, Z., Geizerova, H. and Balcarova, O. Meal frequency and ischemic heart disease. *The Lancet,* 1968, *2*(7561), 190-1.

Fanestil, D. D. and Barrows, C. H., Jr. Aging in the rotifer. *Journal of Gerontology,* 1965, *20*(4), 462-9.

FDA Consumer, Vitamin E, miracle or myth. DHEW Publication 74-20004, 1973. Washington, D.C.: U.S. Government Printing Office.

Finch, C. E. Monamine metabolism in the aging male mouse. In M. Rockstein and M. L. Sussman (Eds.), *Development and Aging of the Nervous System.* New York: Academic Press, 1973, 199.

Finch, C. E. Catecholamine metabolism in the brains of aging mice. In A. N. Norris *et al.* (Eds.) *The Central Nervous System and Aging.* New York: MSS Corporation, 1974, 74-89.

Fineberg, S. K. Evaluation of anorexigenic agents: Studies with chlorphentermine. *American Journal of Clinical Nutrition,* 1962, *11*, 609-16.

Fineberg, S. K. An appraisal of anorexiants in the treatment of obesity. *Journal of the American Geriatric Society,* 1972, *20*(12), 576-9.

Fleck, H. *Introduction to Nutrition.* New York: MacMillan Publishing Company, Inc., 1976.

Fletcher, A. J. A multi-centre study of potassium deficiency in the elderly. *Scottish Medical Journal,* 1974, *19*(3), 142-3.

Food and Nutrition Board, National Research Council. *Recommended Dietary Allowances.* Washington, D.C.: National Academy of Sciences, 1974. 2.

Forbes, G. B. and Reina, J. C. Adult lean body mass declines with age: Some longitudinal observations. *Metabolism: Clinical and Experimental,* 1970, *19*(9), 653-663.

Fox, F. W. The enigma of obesity. *The Lancet,* 1973, *2*(7844) 1487-8.

Freeman, J. T. (Ed.) Nutrition. In *Clinical Features of the Older Patient.* Springfield: Thomas, 1965, 377-89.

Fry, P. C., Fox, H. M. and Linkswiler, H. Nutrient intakes of healthy older women. *Journal of the American Dietetic Association,* 1963, *42*(3), 218-22.

Garn, S. M. Bone loss and aging. In R. Goldman and M. Rockstein (Eds.) *The Physiology and Pathology of Human Aging.* New York: Academic Press, Inc., 1975, 39-58.

Geriatrics. Invisibility of aged may mask scope of malnutrition problem, 1970, *25*(1), 40-44.

Girdwood, R. H., Thomson, A. D. and Williamson, J. Folate status in the elderly. *British Medical Journal,* 1967, *2,* 670-2.

Glanville, E. V., Kaplan, A. R. and Fisher, R. Age, sex, and taste sensitivity. *Journal of Gerontology,* 1964, *19*(4), 474-8.

Glinsman, W. H., Mertz, W. Effect of trivalent chromium on glucose tolerance. Metabolism: Clinical and Experimenta, 1966, *15*(6), 510-20.

Godding, E. W. Dietary fibre redefined. *The Lancet,* 1976, *1*(7969), 1129.

Goldberger, J. and Wheeler, G. A. Experimental pellagra in white male convicts. *Archives of Internal Medicine,* 1920, *25,* 451-71.

Goldrick, R. B., Havenstein, N. and Whyte, H. M. Effect of calories restriction and fenfluramine on weight loss and personality profiles of patients with long standing obesity. *Australian and New Zealand Journal of Medicine,* 1973, *3*(2), 131-141.

Goldstein, J. L., Hazzard, W. R., Schrott, H. G., Bierman, E. L. and Motulsky, A. G. Hyperlipidemia in coronary heart disease I. Lipid levels in 500 survivors of myocardial infarction. *Journal of Clinical Investigation,* 1973a, *52,* 1533.

Goldstein, J. L., Schrott, H. G., Hazzard, W. R., Bierman, E. L. and Motulsky, A. G. Hyperlipidemia in coronary heart disease II. Genetic analysis of lipid levels in 176 families and delineation of a new inherited disorder, combined hyperlipidemia. *Journal of Clinical Investigation,* 1973b, *52,* 1544.

Goodhart, R. S. and Shils, M. E. (Eds.), *Modern Nutrition in Health and Disease.* Philadelphia: Lea & Febiger, 1973, 1153.

Goodman, D. S. and Smith, F. R. Hyperlipidemia, arteriosclerosis and ischemic heart disease. In M. Winick (Ed.), *Nutrition and Aging.* New York: John Wiley and Sons, 1976, 177.

Gordon, P. Free radicals and the aging process. In M. Rockstein, M. L. Sussman and J. Chesky (Eds.), *Theoretical Aspects of Aging.* New York: Academic Press, 1974.

Green, J. Vitamin E and the biological antioxident theory. *Annals of the New York Academy of Science,* 1972, *203,* 29-44.

Greenberg, G. R., Marliss, E. B., Anderson, G. H., Langer, B., Spence, W., Tovee, E. B., and Jeejeebhoy, K. N. Protein-sparing therapy in post operative patients. *New England Journal of Medicine,* 1976, *294*(26), 1411-1416.

Gresham, G. A. Atherosclerosis: Its causes and potential reversibility. *Triangle,* 1976, *15*(2/3), 39-43.

Griffiths, L. L., Brocklehurst, J. C., Scott, D. L., Marks, J. and Blackley, J. Thiamin and ascorbic acid levels in the elderly. *Gerontologia Clinica,* 1967, *9,* 1-10.

Gryfe, C. I., Exton-Smith, A. N., Payne, P. R. and Wheeler, E. F. Pattern of development of bone in childhood adolescence. *The Lancet,* 1971, *1*(7698), 523.

Guth, P. H. Physiologic alterations in small bowel function with age: The absorption of D-xylose. *American Journal of Digestive Diseases,* 1968, *13*(6), 565-71.

Guthrie, H. A. *Introductory Nutrition.* St. Louis: C. V. Mosby Company, 1975, 190-196.

Guthrie, H. A., Black, K. and Madden, J. Nutritional practices of elderly citizens in rural Pennsylvania. *The Gerontologist,* 1972, *12*(4), 330-5.

Gyorgy, P., Cogan, G. and Rose, C. S. Availability of vitamine E in the newborn infant. *Society for Experimental Biology and Medicine, Proceedings,* 1952, *81*(2), 536-8.

Harman, D. Free radical theory of aging: Relations between antiaging and chronic radiation protection agents. *Radiation Research,* 1968a, *35,* 547.

Harman, D. Free radical theory of aging: Effect of free radical reaction inhibitors on mortality rate of male LAF_1 mice. *Journal of Gerontology,* 1968b, *23,* 476-482.

Harman, D. Free radical theory of aging: Effect of the amount and degree of unsaturation of dietary fat on mortality rate. *Journal of Gerontology,* 1971, *26*(4), 451-457.

Harman, D. Free radical theory of aging: Dietary implications. *American Journal of Clinical Nutrition,* 1972, *25,* 839-843.

Harper, A. E. Recommended dietary allowances: Are they what we think they are? In T. P. Labuza (Ed.), *The Nutrition Crisis.* Los Angeles: West Publishing Company, 1975, 22.

Harris, M. Mutation rates in cells at different ploidy levels. *Journal of Cell Physiology,* 1971, *78*(2), 177-184.

Hartshorn, E. A. Food and drug interactions. *Journal of American Dietetics Association,* 1977, *70,* 15.

Hayflick, L. Aging under glass. *Experimental Gerontology,* 1970, *5,* 291.

Hayflick, L. Cell biology of aging. *Bio Science,* 1975, *25*(10), 629-637.

Hazell, K. and Baloch, K. H. Vitamin K deficiency in the elderly. *Gerontologia Clinica,* 1970, *12,* 10-17.

Hazzard, W. R. and Knopp, R. H. Aging and atherosclerosis: Interactions with diet, heredity, and associated risk factors. In T. Rockstein and M. L. Sussman (Eds.), *Nutrition, Longevity, and Aging.* New York: Academic Press, 1976, 143-195.

Heald, F. P. The natural history of obesity. *Advances in Psycholosomatic Medicine (Basel),* 1972, *7,* 102-15.

Hegsted, D. M. Establishment of nutritional requirements in man. *Borden's Review of Nutrition Research,* 1959, *20*(2), 13-22.

Hegsted, D. M. Major minerals. In R. S. Goodhart and M. E. Shils (Eds.), *Modern Nutrition in Health and Disease.* Philadelphia: Lea and Febiger, 1973, 268-286.

Hegsted, D. M. Dietary standards. *Journal of the American Dietetic Association,* 1975a, *66*(1), 13-21.

Hegsted, D. M. Editorial: Dietary standards. *New England Journal of Medicine,* 1975b, *292*(17), 915-7.

Hegsted, D. M. Food and fibre: Evidence from experimental animals. *Nutrition Reviews,* 1977, *35*(3), 45-50.

Henderson, L. M. Nutritional problems growing out of new patterns of food consumption. *American Journal of Public Health,* 1972, *62*(9), 1194-8.

Henkin, R. I., Schecter, P.J., Hoye, R., and Mattern, C. F. T. Ideopathic hypogenia with dysgensea, hyposomia, and dysomia — a new syndrome. *Journal of American Medical Association,* 1971, *217*(4), 434-440.

Henrikson, P. Periodontal disease and calcium deficiency. An experimental study in the dog. *Acta Odontologica Scandinavica,* 1968, *26,* 1.

Herbert, V. Biochemical ane hemotologic lesions in folic acid deficiency. *American Journal of Clinical Nutrition,* 1967, *20*(6), 562-9.

Herbert, V., Folic acid and vitamin B_{12}. In R. S. Goodhart and M. H. Shils (Eds.), *Modern Nutrition in Health and Disease.* Philadelphia: Lea & Febiger, 1973.

Herting, D. C. Perspective on Vitamin E. *American Journal of Clinical Nutrition,* 1966, *19*(3), 210-8.

Hirsch, J. and Knittle, J. L. Cellularity of obese and non-obese human adipose tissue. *Federal Proceedings,* 1970, *29*(4), 1516-21.

Hodkinson, H. M. and Brain, A. T. Unilateral osteoporosis in longstanding hemiplegia in the elderly. *Journal of the American Geriatric Society,* 1967, *15,* 59.

Hodkinson, H. M. Advances in geriatrics. *Practitioner,* 1972, *209,* 513-8.

Hollingsworth, J. W., Bebe, G. W., Ishida, M. and Brill, A. *The uses of vital and health statistics for genetic and radiation studies.* New York: United Nations, Atomic Bomb Casualty Commission, 1962, 77-100.

Holmes, T. and Masuda, M. Psychosomatic Syndrome. *Psychology Today,* 1972, *106,* 71-72.

Hootnick, H. L. Constipation in elderly patients due to drug therapy. *Journal of the American Geriatrics Society,* 1956, *4,* 1021-30.

Hoover, H. C., Grant, J. P., Gorschboth, C. *et al.* Nitrogen-sparing intravenous fluids in postoperative patients. *New England Journal of Medicine,* 1975, *293,* 172-175.

Horwitt, M. K. Niacin-tryptophan relationships in the development of pellagra. *American Journal of Clinical Nutrition,* 1955, *3,* 244-5.

Horwitt, M. K., Harvey, C. C., Duncan, G. D. and Wilson, W. C. Effects of limited tocopherol intake in man with relationships to erythrocyte hemolysis and lipid oxidations. *American Journal of Clinical Nutrition,* 1956, *4*(4), 408-19.

Hruza, Z. and Hlavachova, V. The characteristics of newly formed collagen during aging. *Gerontology,* 1963, *7,* 221-232.

Hughes, G. Changes in taste sensitivity with advancing age. *Gerontologia Clinica,* 1969, *11*(4), 224-30.

Hurdle, A. D. F. and Williams, T. C. Picton, folic-acid deficiency in elderly patients admitted to hospital. *British Medical Journal,* 1966, *2*(5507), 202-5.

Hurxthal, L. M. and Vose, G. P. The relationship of dietary calcium intake to radiographic bone density in normal and osteoporotic persons. *Calcified Tissue Research* (Berlin), 1969, *4,* 245.

Hyams, D. E. The absorption of vitamin B_{12} in the elderly. *Gerontologia Clinica,* 1964, *6,* 193-206.

Hyams, D. E. Nutrition of the elderly. *Modern Geriatrics,* 1973, *3*(7), 352-9.

Inoue, T., Sakakida, H., and Katsura, E. Energy requirements in the aged. *Acta Scholae Medicinalis Universitatis (Kioto),* 1962, *38,* 227-32.

Irwin, M. and Feeley, R. M. Frequency and size of meals and serum lipids, nitrogen and mineral retention, fat digestibility, and urinary thiamine and riboflavin in young women. *American Journal of Clinical Nutrition,* 1967, *20*(8), 816-24.

Irwin, M. I. and Hegsted, D. M. A conspectus of research on protein requirements of a man. *Journal of Nutrition,* 1971, *101*(3), 385-429.

Irwin, M. J. and Hutchens, B. K. A conspectus of research on vitamin requirements of man. *Journal of Nutrition,* 1976, *106*(6), 821-879.

Isaacs, B. Can this new diet prevent heart attacks? *New York,* 1976, *9*(45), 48-51.

Ivy, A. C., Grossman, M. I. Digestive system. In *Cowdry's Problems of Aging: Biological and Medical Aspects.* Baltimore: Williams & Wilkins, 1952, 497-9.

Jacobs, A. and Greeman, D. A. Availability of food iron. *British Medical Journal,* 1969, *1,* 673-6.

Joint FAO/WHO Expert Committee on Trace Elements in Human Nutrition. *Trace Elements in Human Nutrition.* Geneva: WHO Technical Report Series, 1973, 532.

Jones, J. E., Shane, S. R., Jacobs, W. H. and Flink, E. B. Magnesium balance studies in chronic alcoholism. *Annals of New York Academy of Science,* 1969, *162,* 934.

Joske, R. A. Finckh, E. S. and Wood, I. J. Gastric biopsy: Study of 1000 consecutive successful gastric biopsies. *Quarterly Journal of Medicine,* 1955, *24,* 269-94.

Joske, R. A., Shamma, M. H. and Drummey, G. D. Intestinal malabsorption following temporary occlusion of the superior mesenteric artery. *American Journal of Medicine,* 1958, *25,* 449.

Jowsey, J. Prevention and treatment of osteoporosis. In M. Winick (Ed.), *Nutrition and Aging.* New York: John Wiley and Sons, 1976, 131.

Judge, T. G. Potassium metabolism in the elderly. In L. A. Carlson, (Ed.), *Nutrition in Old Age,* Symposium Swedish Nutrition Foundation, Uppsala, 1972, *10,* 86-99.

Judge, T. G. The milieu interieur and aging. In J. C. Brocklehurst (Ed.), *Textbook of Geriatric Medicine and Gerontology.* London: Churchill Livingstone, 1973, 113-121.

Judge, T. G. and Cowan, N. R. Dietary potassium intake and grip strength in older people. *Gerontologia Clinica (Switzerland)* 1971, *13*(4), 221-6.

Kallman, F. J. and Jarvick, L. Individual differences in constitution and genetic background. In J. E. Birren (Ed.) *Handbook of Aging and the Individual.* Chicago: University of Chicago Press, 1959, 216-263.

Kallstrom, B. and Nyloff, R. Vitamin B_{12} and folic acid in psychiatric disorders. *Acta Psychiatrica Scandinavica*

(Denmark), 1969, *45*(2), 137-152.

Kannel, W. B. and Gordon, T. Obesity and cardiovascular disease. The Framingham study. In W. L. Burland, P. D. Samuel and J. Yudkin (Eds.), *Obesity Symposium.* Edinburgh: Livingstone, 1973, 24-51, 57-59.

Kaplan, A. R., Glanville, E. V. and Fischer, R. Cumulative effect of age and smoking on taste sensitivity in males and females. *Journal of Gerontology,* 1965, *20,* 334.

Kataria, M. S., Rao, D. B. and Curtis, R. C. Vitamin C levels in the elderly. *Gerontologia Clinica,* 1965, *7,* 189.

Kay, R. M. and Truswell, A. S. The effect of wheat fibre on the plasma cholesterol in rats. *Procedures in Nutrition Society,* 1975, *34,* 17A.

Kay, M. M. B., and Makinodan, T. Immunobiology of aging: Evaluation of current status. *Clinical Immunology and Immunopathology,* 1976, *6,* 394-413.

Kelley, L., Ohlson, M. A. and Harper, L. J. Food selection and well being in aging women. *Journal of the American Dietetic Association,* 1957, *33,* 466.

Keusch, G. T., Troncale, F. J. and Plant, A. G. Neomycin-induced malabsorption in a tropical population. *Gastrenterology,* 1970, *58,* 197-202.

Khan, R. M., Hodge, J. S., and Bassett, H. F. Magnesium in open-heart surgery. *Journal of Thoracic and Cardiovascular Surgery,* 1973 *66*(2), 185-91.

Kiehm, T. G., Anderson, J. W. and Ward, K. Beneficial effects of a high carbohydrate, high-fiber diet on hyperglycemic diabetic men. *American Journal of Clinical Nutrition,* 1976, *29,* 899.

Kimura, K. K. Refine carbohydrates, dietary fiber, and gastrointestinal abnormality. *Journal of American Medical Association,* 1976, *235,* 375.

Kirk, J. E. and Chieffi, M. Hypovitaminemia A: Effect of Vitamin A administration on plasma vitamin A concentration, conjunctual changes, dark adaptation and toad skin. *American Journal of Clinical Nutrition,* 1952, *1*(1), 37-43.

Klevay, L. M. Coronary heart disease: The zinc/copper hypothesis, *American Journal of Clinical Nutrition,* 1975, *28,* 764-774.

Krieger, A. Production and acceptance of low-calorie foods. *Bibleotheca Nutrito et Dieta,* 1973, *18,* 171-8.

Labuza, T. P. *The Nutrition Crisis: A Reader.* St. Paul: West Publishing Co., 1975, 102.

Labuza, T. P. *Food and Your Well Being.* Los Angeles: West Publishing Co., 1977, 104.

Lamb, M. J. and Maynard-Smith, J. Radiation and aging in insects. *Experimental Gerontology,* 1964, *1,* 11-20.

Latchford, W. Nutritional problems of the elderly. *Community Health,* 1974, *6*(3), 145-149.

Lea, A. J. Dietary factors associated with death-rates from certain neoplasmas in man. *The Lancet,* 1966, *2*(7458), 332-3.

Leaf, A. Getting old. *Scientific American,* 1973, *229*(3), 28-36.

Lear, J. The flimsy staff of life. *Saturday Review,* 1970, *53*(4) 53-54.

LeBovit, C and Baker, D. A. Food consumption and dietary levels of older households in Rochester, New York. *Home Economics Research Report.* Washington, D.C.: U.S. Department of Agriculture, 1965, (25).

Lennart, L. (Ed.) *Emotions: Their Parameter and Measurement.* New York: Raven Press Publishers.

Leon, G. R. Treatment of obesity. A behavior modification approach. *Minnesota Medicine,* 1974, *57*(12), 977-80.

Leon, G. R. and Chamberlain, K. Emotional arousal, eating patterns and body image as differential factors associated with varying success in maintaining a weight loss. *Journal of Consulting and Clinical Psychology,* 1973a, *40,* 474.

Leon, G. R. and Chamberlain, K. A comparison of daily eating habits and emotional states of overweight persons successful and unsuccessful in maintaining a weight loss. *Journal of Consulting and Clinical Psychology,* 1973b, *41,* 108.

Leonard, J. N., Hofer, J. L., Pritikin, N. *Live Longer Now,* New York: Grosset and Dunlap, 1974.

Lepshitz, D. A., Bothwell, T. H., Seftel, H. C., Wapnick, A. A. and Chareton, R. W. The role of ascorbic acid in the metabolism of storage iron. *British Journal of Haematology,* 1971, *20,* 155-163.

180   *Appendix II*

Levander, O. A. Selenium and chromium in human nutrition. *American Dietetic Association Journal,* 1975, *66*(4), 338-44.

Leverton, R. M. The RDAs are not for amateurs. *American Dietetic Association Journal,* 1975, *66*(1), 9-11.

Levi, L. *Society, Stress and Disease.* London: Oxford University Press, 1971.

Levi, L. (Ed.) Emotions: Their Parameters and Measurement. New York: Raven Press, 1975.

Levin, B. Quoted in Food and Nutrition News, 1977, *48*(4), 2.

Levine, R. H., Streeten, D. H. P. and Doisy, R. J. Effects of oral chromium supplementation on the glucose tolerance of elderly human subjects. *Metabolism: Clinical and Experimental (N.Y.)* 1968, *17*(2), 114-25.

Levrat, M., Pasquier, J., Lambert, R., *et al.* Peptic ulcer in patients over 60. *American Journal of Digestive Diseases,* 1966, *11,* 279.

Li, T. K. and Vallee, B. Biochemical and nutritional role of trace elements. In R. S. Goodhart and M. E. Shils (Eds.), *Modern Nutrition in Health and Disease,* Philadelphia: Lea and Febiger, 1973.

Liang, P. H., Hil, T. T., Jan, O. H., and Grok, L. T. Evaluation of mental development in relation to early malnutrition. *American Journal of Clinical Nutrition,* 1967, *20,* 1290.

Lim, P. and Jacob, E. Magnesium deficiency in patients on longterm diuretic therapy for heart failure. *British Medical Journal,* 1972, *3,* 620-2.

Linkwiler, H., Joyce, C. L., Anand, C. R. Calcium retention of young adult males as affected by level of protein and of calcium intake. *Transactions of the New York Academy of Sciences.* Series II, Vol. 36(4), 1074, 333-340.

Lloyd, E. L. Serum iron levels and haematological status in the elderly. *Gerontologica Clinica (Basel),* 1971, *13,* 246-55.

Long, R. Y. Cancer: Nutritional deficiency disease. *Journal of Applied Nutrition,* 1976, *28*(3 & 4), 5-20.

Lotz, M., Zisman, E., and Barrter, F. C. Evidence for a phosphorous depletion syndrome in man. *New England*

Journal of Medicine, 1968, *278,* 409-415.

Lutwak, L. Osteoporosis: A mineral deficiency disease. *Journal of the American Dietetic Association,* 1964, *44,* 173.

Lutwak, L. Effects of estrogens and androgens in metabolic bone disease. *2nd International Congress of Hormonal Steroids,* 1966, 326.

Lutwak, L. Nutritional aspects of osteoporsis. Symposium on osteoporosis. *American Geriatrics Society Journal,* 1969, *17*(2), 115-119.

Lutwak, L., Krook, L., Henrikson, P. A., Uris, R., Whalen, J., Coulston, A. and Lesser, G. Calcium deficiency and human periodontal disease. *Israel Journal of Medical Science,* 1971, *7,* 504.

Lutwak, L. Dietary calcium and the reversal of bone demineralization. *Nutrition News,* 1974, *37*(1), 1-4.

Lutwak, L. Dietary calcium and the reversal of bone demineralization. In T. R. Labuza (Ed.) *The Nutrition Crisis.* Los Angeles: West Publishing Company, 1975, 201-204.

Lutwak, L. Periodontal disease. In M. Winick (Ed.), *Nutrition and Aging.* New York: John Wiley and Sons, 1976, 145.

MacDonald, M. T. Diet and human atherosclerosis . . . carbohydrates. *Advances in Experimental Medicine and Biology,* 1975, *60,* 57-64.

MacDonald, M. T. and Stewart, J. B. Nutrition and low-income families. *Proceedings of the Nutrition Society,* 1974, *33,* 75-78.

Mack, P. B., LaChance, P. A., Vose, G. P. and Vogt, F. B. Bone demineralization of foot and hand of Gemini-Titan IV, V, and VII astronauts during orbital flight. *American Journal of Roentgenology, Radium Therapy and Nuclear Medicine,* 1967, *C*(3), 503.

MacLennan, W. J., Andrews, G. R., MacLeod, C. and Caird, F. I. Anaemia in the elderly. *Quarterly Journal of Medicine (Oxford),* 1973, *42,* 1-13.

MacLeod, C. C., Judge, T. G. and Caird, F. I. Nutrition of the elderly at home, II: Intakes of vitamins. *Age and Aging,* 1974, *3*(4), 209-20.

MacLeod, C. C., Judge, T. G. and Caird, F. I. Nutrition of

the elderly at home, III: Intakes of minerals. *Age and Aging,* 1975, *4*(1), 49-57.

Mahoney, M. J. Self-reward and self-monitoring techniques for weight control. *Behavior Research and Therapy (Oxford),* 1974, *5,* 48.

Majaj, A. S., Dinning, J. S., Ozzam, S. A. and Darby, W. J. Vitamin E responsive megaloblastic anemia in infants with protein-caloric malnutrition. *American Journal of Clinical Nutrition,* 1963, *12,* 374-9.

Makinodan, T. Immunity and aging. In C. L. Finch and L. Hayflick, (Eds.), *Handbook of the Biology of Aging.* San Francisco: Van Nostrand Reinhold Company, 1977, 379-402.

Makinodan, T. and Adler, W. H. Effects of aging on the differentiation and proliferation potentials of cells of the immune system. *Federal Proceedings,* 1975, *34,* 153-158.

Manavsos, O. N., Truelove, S. C., and Lumsden, K. Prevalence of colonic diverticulosis in general population of Oxford area. *British Medical Journal,* 1967, *3,* 762-3.

Mann, G. V. Relationship of age to nutritional requirements. *American Journal of Clinical Nutrition,* 1973, *26*(10), 1096-7.

Mann, G. V. and Spoerry, A. Studies of a surfactant and cholesteremia in the Masai. *American Journal of Clinical Nutrition,* 1974, *27*(5), 464-469.

March, D. C. *Handbook: Interactions of Selected Drugs with Nutritional Status in Man.* Chicago: The American Dietetic Association, 1976.

Marks, J. Nutrition of the elderly: Present and future research. *Royal Society for the Promotion of Health Journal* (London), 1969, *89*(6), 289-92.

Martin, G. M., Sprague, C. A. and Epstein, C. J. Replicative lifespan of cultivated human cells: Effect of donor's age, tissue and genotype. *Laboratory Investigation,* 1970, *23,* 86-92.

Mayer, J. Regulation of energy intake and the body weight: The glucostatic theory and the lipstatic hypothesis. *Annals of the New York Academy of Science,* 1955, *63,* 15-43.

Mayer, J. Treatment of obesity in adults. *Postgraduate Medicine,* 1965, *38,* A-133.

Mayer, J. *Overweight: Causes, Costs and Control.* Englewood Cliffs, New Jersey: Prentice-Hall, Inc., 1968.

Mayer, J. Aging and nutrition. *Geriatrics,* 1974, *29*(5), 57-9.

Mayer, J. *A Diet for Living.* New York: David McKay Co., Inc., 1975a, 50-51.

Mayer, J. Quoted in R. Butler (Ed.) *Why Survive? Being Old in America.* San Francisco: Harper and Row Publishers, 1975b, 366.

McCay, C. M. Nutritional aspects of aging. *Old Age in the Modern World.* London: Livingstone, 1955.

McCay, C. M., Crowell, M. F. and Maynard, L. A. The effect of retarded growth upon the length of lifespan and upon the ultimate body size. *Journal of Nutrition,* 1935, *10,* 63-79.

McCracken, B. H. Etiological aspects of obesity. In A. M. Lilienfeld and A. J. Gifford (Eds.), *Chronic Diseases and Public Health,* Baltimore: Johns Hopkins Press, 1966, 125-37.

McCuish, A. G., Munro, J. F. and Duncan, L. J. P. Follow-up study of refractory obesity, treated by fasting. *British Medical Journal,* 1968, *1,* 91.

Mehta, S. K., Wesser, E. and Sleisenger, M. A. The in vitro effects of bacterial metabolites and antibotics in pancreatic lipase activity. *Journal of Clinical Investigation,* 1964, *43,* 1252.

Mertin, J. Letter: Polyunsaturated fatty acids and cancer. *British Medical Journal,* 1973, *4,* 357.

Mertz, W. Biological role of chromium. *Federation Proceedings,* 1967, *26,* 186-93.

Michelmore, P. A model geriatric health care system. *Geriatrics,* 1975, *30*(2), 146-154.

Miller, D. S. and Payne, P. R. Longevity and protein uptake. *Experimental Gerontology,* 1968, *3,* 231-234.

Miller, J. M. and Stare, F. J. Nutritional problems and dietary requirements. In T. H. Powers (Ed.), *Surgery of the Aged and Debilitated Patients.* Philadelphia: Saunders, 1968, 123-37.

Miller, O. N., Hamilton, J. G. and Goldsmith, G. A. Investigation of the mechanism of action of nicotinic acid on serum lipid levels in man. *American Journal of C linical Nutrition,* 1960, *8*(4), 480-90.

Milne, J. S., Lonegran, M. E., Williamson, J., *et al.* Leucocyte ascorbic acid levels and vitamin C intake in older people. *British Medical Journal,* 1971, *4,* 383-6.

Mitra, M. L. Vitamin C deficiency in the elderly and its manifestations. *Acta Gerontologica et Geriatrica Belgica (Belgium),* 1969, *7, 65-7.*

Mitra, M. L. Confusional states in relation to vitamin deficiencies in the elderly. *Journal of the American Geriatrics Society,* 1971, *19*(6), 536-45; also in *Acta Gerontologica et Geriatrica Belgica (Belgium),* 1970, *8,* 103-6.

Modell, W. States and prospect of drugs and overeating. *Journal of the American Medical Association,* 1960, *173,* 1131-6.

Modell, W. Symposium: Use of drugs in the elderly patient. *Geriatrics,* 1974, *29,* 50.

Moment, G. B. The Ponce de Leon trail today. *Bio Science,* 1975, *25*(10), 623-628.

Montoye, H. J., Epstein, F. H. and Kjelsberg, M. O. Relationship between serum cholesterol and body fatness. An epidemiologic study. *American Journal of Clinical Nutrition,* 1966, *18,* 397-407.

Moore, C. V. Iron nutrition and requirements. *Scandinavian Journal of Haemetology.* Series Haematologica 6, 1965, 1-13.

Moore, C. V. Iron. In R. S. Goodhart and M. E. Shils (Eds.), *Modern Nutrion in Health and Disease: Diet Therapy.* Philadelphia: Lea and Febiger, 1973, 300-301.

Moore, F. D., Lester, J., Boyden, C. M., Ball, M. R., Sullivan, N., and Dagher, F. J. The skeleton as a feature of body composition: Values predicted by isotope dilution and observed by cadaver dissection in adult human female. *Human Biology,* 1968, *40,* 135.

Moore, Ball, M. R. and Boyden, C. M. *The Body Cell Mass and its Supporting Environment.* Philadelphia: W. B. Saunders, 1963.

Morgan, A. F. Nutritional status, U.S.A. *California Agricultural Experiment Station Bulletin (Berkeley, California),* 1959, *769,* 81.

Morgan, A. F. Nutrition of the aging. *The Gerontologist,* 1962, *2*(2), 77-84.

Morgan, A. F., Gillum, H. L. and Williams, B. I. Nutritional status of the aging: 3: Serum ascorbic acid and intake. *Journal of Nutrition,* 1955, *55,* 431.

Morgan, A. F., Wales, M. B., Pulvertaft, C. N. and Fourman, P. Effects of age on the loss of bone after gastric surgery. *The Lancet,* 1966, *1*(7467), 772-6.

Morson, B. C. The muscle abnormality of diverticular disease of the sigmoid colon. *British Journal of Radiology,* 1963, *36,* 385.

Moss, G. E. *Illness, Immunity and Social Interaction: The Dynamics of Biosocial Resonation.* New York: John Wiley and Sons, Inc., 1973.

Munro, H. N. Protein requirements and metabolism in aging. In L. A. Carlson (Ed.), *Nutrition in Old Age.* Uppsala, Sweden: Swedish Nutrition Foundation, 1972, 32-54.

Munro, H. N. Report of a conference on protein and amino acid needs for growth and development. *American Journal of Clinical Nutrition,* 1974, *27*(1), 55-58.

Murphy, F., Srvastava, P. C., Varadi, S. and Elwis, A. Screening of psychiatric patients for hypovitaminosis B_{12}. *British Medical Journal,* 1969, *3,* 559-60.

National Center for Health Statistics. *Need for Dental Care Among Adults, U.S. 1960-1962.* Washington, D.C.: United States Department of Health, Education and Welfare, Public Health Service, Series II, 1970 (36).

Nelson, R. A. Quoted from newspaper report of comments at the 4th Annual Nutrition Conference of Dairy Council of California. *Los Angeles Times,* April 25, 1974, Part VI, 1,8.

Nelson, R. A., Anderson, L. E., Gastineau, C. F. Hayles, A. B. and Stamnes, C. L. Physiology and natural history of obesity. *Journal of the American Medical Association,* 1973, *223*(6), 627-30.

Newton-John, J. R. and Morgan, D. B. Osteoporosis: Disease or senescence? *The Lancet,* 1968, *1*(7536), 232-3.

Ng, C. W. Poznanski, W. J., Borowecki, M. Reimer, G. Differences in growth in vitro of adipose cells from normal and obese patients. *Nature,* 1971, *231* (5303), 445.

Noble, I. T. A study of food behavior of a selected elderly population as related to socio-economic and psychologic factors. *Dissertation Abstracts,* 1969, *29*(8-B), 2952.

Noble, R. E. A controlled study of a weight reduction regimen. *Current Therapeutic Research (Clinical & Experimental)* (U.S.) 1971, *13*, 685-91.

Nordin, B. E. C. Osteomalacia, osteoporosis and calcium deficiency. *Clinical Orthopaedics & Related Research,* 1960, *17*, 235.

Nordin, B. E. C., Aaron, J., Gallagher, J. C. and Horsman, A. Calcium and bone metabolism in old age. In L. A. Carlson (Ed.) *Nutrition in Old Age.* Uppsala: Symposium Swedish Nutrition Foundation, 1972, *10,* 77-84.

Novak, L. P. Aging, total body potassium, fat-free mass and cell mass in males and females between ages 18-85 years. *Journal of Gerontology,* 1972, *27*(4), 438.

Nutrition News. Role of dietary calcium in human periodontal disease. Graduate School, Cornell University, 1970.

Nutrition Reviews. On meeting certain recommended dietary allowances in the elderly and indolent, 1966, *24,* 319.

Nutrition Reviews. Diet and cancer of the colon, 1973, *31*(4), 110-1.

Nutrition Reviews. 5th Annual Marabou Symposium — Food and Fiber, 1977, *35*(3), 71-72.

Ohlson, M. A. Food for the aging. *Medical Times (London),* 1964, *92,* 879-84.

Oscancova, K. and Hejda, S. Nutrition and attitude to obesity. Epidemiological survey in a population with a high prevalence of obesity. *Review of Czechoslovak Medicine (Praha),* 1970, *16*(3), 131-9.

Osborn, M. O. Nutrition of the aged. In A. M. Hoffman (Ed.), *The Daily Needs and Interests of Older People.* Springfield: Thomas, 1970, 235-57.

Orgell, L. E. Aging of clones of mamalian cells. *Nature,* 1973, *243,* 441-445.

Packer, L., Deamer, D. W., and Heath, R. L. Regulation and deterioration of structure in membranes. *Advances in Gerontological Research,* 1967, *2,*108.

Painter, N. S., Almeida, A. Z. and Colebourne, K. W. Unprocessed bran in treatment of diverticular disease of the colon. *British Medical Journal,* 1972, *2,* 137.

Painter, N. S., Burkitt, D. P. Diverticular disease of the colon: A deficiency disease of western civilization. *British Medical Journal,* 1971, *2,* 450, 654, 707-8, 772.

Pao, E. Food patterns of the elderly. *Family Economics Review,* 1971, 16.

Passmore, R. *et al. Handbook on Human Nutritional Requirements.* FAO Nutritional Studies. Geneva: WHO, 1974 (61).

Pawan, Gl L. S. Drugs and appetite. *Proceedings of Nutrition Society,* 1974, *33,* 239-244.

Pearce, M. L. and Dayton, S. Incidence of cancer in men on a diet high in polyunsaturated fat. *The Lancet,* 1971, *1*(7697), 464-7.

Petersen, D. M. and Whittington, F. J. Drug use among the elderly: A review. *Journal of Psychedelic Drugs,* 1977, *9*(1), 25-37.

Phillips, R. L. Role of life-style and dietary habit on risk of cancer among Seventh-day Adventists. *Cancer Research,* 1975, *35,* 3513.

Pollack, H. Malnutrition. In W. T. Marxer and G. R. Cowgill (Eds.), *The Art of Predictive Medicine.* Springfield: Thomas, 1967, 104-8.

Pories, W. J., Henzel, J. H., Rob, C. C. and Strain, W. H. Acceleration of wound healing in man with zinc sulphate given by mouth. *The Lancet,* 1967, *1*(482), 121-124.

Portis, S. A. & King, J. C. The gastrointestinal tract of the aged. *Journal of the American Medical Association,* 1952, *148,* 1073-79.

Pridie, K. B. Incidence and coincidence of hiatus hernia. *Gut,* 1966, *7,* 188-9.

Pritikin, N., Kern, J., Prihkin, R. and Kaye, S. M. Diet and exercise as a total therapeutic regimen for the rehabilitation of patients with severe peripheral vascular disease. Atlanta: 52nd Annual Session of the American Congress on Rehabilitation Medical, 1975.

Pullen, F. W. II. Pories, W. J. and Strain, W. H. Delayed healing: The rationale for zinc therapy. *Laryngoscope (U.S.),* 1971, *81*(10), 1638-49.

Pyke, D. A. Aetiological factors. In W. G. Oakley, D. A. Pyke, and K. W. Taylor (Eds.), *Clinical Diabetes and its Biochemical Basis.* Oxford, England: Blackwell Scientific Publications, 1968.

Rafsky, H. A., Newman, B. Vitamin B excretion in the aged. *Gastroenterology,* 1943, *1,* 737.

Rafsky, H. A. and Newman, B. A study of vitamin A and carotene tolerance tests in the aged. *Gastroenterology,* 1948, *10,*

Rahe, R., McKean, J. D. and Ransom, A. J. A longitudinal study of life changes and illness patterns. *Journal of Psychosomatic Research,* 1967, *10,* 355-66.

Rahe, H., Mahan, J. and Arthur, R. J. Predictions of near future health; change from subjects preceeding life change. *Journal of Psychosomatic Research,* 1970, *14,* 401-406.

Randall, R. E. Magnesium metabolism in chronic renal disease. *Annals of New York Academy of Science,* 1969, *162,* 831.

Ranhotra, G. S. Effect of cellulose and wheat millfractions on plasma and liver cholesterol in cholesterol fed rats. *Cereal Chemistry,* 1973, *50,* 358.

Rao, D. B. Problems of nutrition in the aged. Journal of the *American Geriatrics Society,* 1973, *21*(8), 362-7.

Read, A. E., Gough, K. R., Pardoe, J. R. and Nicholas, A. Nutritional studies on the entrants to an old people's home, with particular reference to folic-acid deficiency. *British Medical Journal,* 1965, *2,* 843-8.

Regnier, E. The administration of large doses of ascorbic acid in the prevention and treatment of the common cold. Part I. *Review of Allergy: Selected Abstracts of Allergology,* 1968, *22*(9), 835-46.

Regnier, E. The administration of large doses of ascorbic acid in the prevention and treatment of the common cold, Part II. *Review of Allergy: Selected Abstracts of Allergology,* 1968, *22*(10), 948-56.

Riccitelli, M. L. Vitamin C therapy in geriatric practice.

Journal of the American Geriatrics Society, 1972, *20*(1), 34-42.

Richter, C. P. and Campbell, K. H. Sucrose taste thresholds of rats and humans. *American Journal of Physiology,* 1940, *128,* 291-8.

Riggs, B. C., Jowsey, J., Goldsmith, R. S., Kelly, P. J., Hoffman, D. L., and Arnaud, C. D. Short and long-term effects of estrogen and synthetic anabolic hormone in postmenopausal osteoporosis. *Journal of Clinical Investigation,* 1972, *51,* 1659-1663.

Rimm, A. A., Werner, L. H., Yserloo, B. and Bernstein, R. A. Relationship of obesity and disease in 73,532 weight-conscious women. *Public Health Reports,* 1975, *90*(1), 44-51.

Rivlin, R. S. Riboflavin metabolism. *New England Journal of Medicine,* 1970, *283*(9), 463-72.

Robertson, L., Flinders, C., Godfrey, B. *Laurel's Kitchen.* Berkeley: Nilgiri Press, 1976, 434-437.

Robinson, C. H. Fluid and electrolyte balance. *Normal and Therapeutic Nutrition.* New York: Macmillan Company, 1972, 125-144.

Robson, J. R. K. in collaboration with F. A. Larkin, A. M. Sandretto, and B. Tadayyon. *Malnutrition Causation and Control.* New York: Gordon Breach Science Publications, Inc., 1972.

Rockstein, M. Molecular genetic mechanisms in development and aging. In M. Rockstein and G. T. Baker (Eds.), *Symposium on Molecular Genetic Mechanisms in Development and Aging.* New York: Academic Press, 1972.

Ranhotra, G. S. Effect of cellulose and wheat mill fractions on plasma and liver cholesterol in cholesterol fed rats. *Cereal Chemistry,* 1973, *50,* 358.

Roe, D. A. *Drug Induced Nutritional Deficiencies.* Westport, Connecticut: Avi Publishing Company, Inc. 1976.

Rose, G. A. Study of the treatment of osteoporosis with fluroide therapy and high calcium intake. *Proceedings of the Royal Society of Medicine,* 1965, *58,* 436.

Rose, G. A. Clinical aspects of calcium metabolism bone disease. *Transactions of the Medical Society of London,* 1970, *86,* 62.

Rose, G., Blackburn, H., Keys, A., Taylor, H. L., Kannel, W. B., Paul, O., Reid, D. O. and Stamler, J. Colon cancer and blood-cholesterol. *The Lancet,* 1974, *1*(7850), 181-3.

Ross, M. H. Nutrition, disease and length of life. In G. E. W. Wolstenholme & M. O'Connor (Eds.) *Diet and Bodily Constitution.* Boston: Little, Brown, Ciba Foundation Study Group, 1964, (17), 90-103.

Ross, M. H. Length of life and caloric intake. *American Journal of Clinical Nutrition,* 1972, *25,* 834.

Ross, M. H. and Bras, G. Lasting influence of early caloric restriction on prevalence of neoplasms in the rat. *U.S. National Cancer Institute Journal,* 1971, *47*(50), 1095-1113.

Ross, M. H. and Bras, G. Dietary preference and diseases of age. *Nature,* 1974, *250,* 834.

Roundtree, J. L. and Tinklin, G. L. Food beliefs and practices of selected senior citizens. *Gerontologist,* 1975, *15*(6), 537-540.

Ryder, J. B. Steatorrhea in the elderly. *Gerontologia Clinica,* 1963, *5* 1), 30.

Sacher, G. A. Molecular versus systemic theories on genesis of aging. *Experimental Gerontology,* 1968, *3,* 265-271.

Sacks, F. M., Castelli, W. P., Donner, A. and Kass, E. H. Plasma lipids and lipoproteins in vegetarians and controls. *New England Journal of Medicine,* 1975, *292*(22), 1148-1151.

Sahud, M. A. Update and reduction of dehydriascorbic acid in human platelets. *Clinical Research,* 1970, *18,* 133.

Salans, L. B., Cushman, W. S., Weismann, R. E. Studies of human adipose tissue. Adipose cell size and number in non-obese and obese patients. *Journal of Clinical Investigation,* 1973, *42,* 929-941.

Scala, J. Fiber, the forgotten nutrient. *Food Technology,* 1974, *28,* 34-6.

Schlenker, E. D., Feurig, J. S., Stone, L. H., Ohlson, M. A. and Mickelsen, O. Nutrition and health of older people. *American Journal of Clinical Nutrition,* 1973, *26*(10), 1111-9.

Schlettwein-Gsell, D. Nutrition as a factor in aging. In N. W. Shock, (Ed.), *Perspectives in Experimental Gerontology,*

Springfield; Thomas, 1966, 280-6.

Schneider, H. A. and Hesla, J. T. The way it is. *Nutrition Reviews,* 1973, *31*(8), 233-7.

Schroeder, H. A. Nutrition. In E. V. Dowdry, F. U. Steinberg (Eds.) *The Care of the Geriatric Patient.* St. Louis: Mosby, 1971, 137-61.

Schroeder, H. A., Nason, A. P. and Tipton, I. H. Essential trace metals in man: Cobalt. *Journal of Chronic Diseases (U.S.)* 1967, *20,* 869-90.

Schroeder, H. A., Nason, A. P., Tipton, I. H. Essential metals in man, magnesium. *Journal of Chronic Disease,* 1969, *21,* 815.

Scrimshaw, N. S. Synergistic and antagonistic interactions of nutrition and infection. *Federation Proceedings,* 1966, *25*(6) Part I, 1679-1681.

Scrimshaw, N. S. Nutrition and stress. In G. E. W. Wolstenholme and M. O'Connor (Eds.) *Diet and Bodily Constitution.* Boston: Little Brown: Ciba Foundation Study Group, 1964 (17), 40-54.

Sebrell, W. H., Jr. It's not age that interferes with nutrition of the elderly. *Nutrition Today,* 1966, *1,* 15-18.

Sebrell, W. H. and Haggerty, J. J. *Food and Nutrition.* New York: Time Life Books, 1967, 11.

Seeling, M. S. The requirement of magnesium by the normal adult. *American Journal of Clinical Nutrition,* 1964, *14,* 342.

Selye, H. A. Stress and aging. *Journal of the American Geriatrics Society,* 1970, *18*(9), 669-690.

Shawver, J. R., Scarborough, J. S. and Tarnowski, S. M. Control of hypercholesteremia and hyperlipemia in a neuropsychiatric hospital. *American Journal of Psychiatry,* 1961, *117,* 741-2.

Shils, M. E. Experimental production of magnesium deficiency in man. *Annals of the New York Academy of Science,* 1969, *162,*(2), 847-55.

Shils, M. E. Nutrition and neoplasia. In R. S. Goodhart and M. E. Shils (Eds.), *Modern Nutrition in Health and Disease.* Philadelphia: Lea & Febiger, 1973.

Shock, N. W. Physiological theories of aging. In M. Rockstein, M. Sussman and J. Chevsky (Eds.), *Theoretical*

Aspects of Aging. New York: Academic Press, 1974, 119-136.

Silberberg, M. and Silberberg, R. Diet and lifespan. *Physiological Review,* 1955, *35*(2), 347-62.

Silink, S. J., Nobile, S., and Woodhill, J. M. Clinical and biochemical assessment of nutritional status. *Modern Nutrition,* 1973, *3*(7), 366-74.

Simonson, E. and Keys, A. Research in Russia on vitamins and atherosclerosis. *Circulation,* 1961, *24,* 1239-48.

Sims, E. A. H., Horton, E. S. and Salans, B. The inducible metabolic abnormalities during development of obesity. *Annual Review of Medicine,* 1971, *22,* 235-250.

Sinclair, H. M. Assessment and results of obesity. *British Medical Journal,* 1953, *2,* 1404-7.

Sinex, M. The programmed theory of aging. In M. Rockstein, M. Sussman and J. Chevsky (Eds.), *Theoretical Aspects of Aging.* New York: Academic Press, 1974, 23-32.

Sklar, M. Functional gastrointestinal disease in the aged. *American Journal of Gastroenterology,* 1970, *53,* 570.

Smith, D. W. and Bierman, E. L. (Eds.), *The Biologic Ages of Man.* Philadelphia: W. B. Saunders Co., 1973, 154-190.

Smith, R. W., Rizek, J. and Frame, B. Determinants of serum antirachitic activity. Special reference to involutional osteoporosis. *American Journal of Clinical Nutrition,* 1964, *14,* 98-108.

Smith, R. W. and Rizek, J. Epidemiologic studies of osteoporosis in women of Puerto Rico and southeastern Michigan with special reference to age, race, national origin, and to other related or associated findings. *Clinical Orthopaedics and Related Research,* 1966, *45,* 31.

Smith, S. G. and Martin, D. W. Cheilosis successfully treated with synthetic vitamin B_6. Society for *Experimental Biology and Medicine, Proceedings,* 1940, *43,* 660-3.

Sohar, E. and Sneh, E. Follow-up of obese patients: 14 years after a successful reducing diet. *American Journal of Clinical Nutrition,* 1973, *26*(8), 845-8.

Solomon, N. The study and treatment of the obese patient. *Hospital Practice,* 1969, *4*(3), 90-94.

Somogyi, J. C. Prevention of atherosclerosis by diet. Present status and conclusions. *Advances in Experimental Medicine and Biology,* 1975, *60,* 205-230.

Spies, T. D., Bean, W. B. and Ashe, W. F. A note on the use of vitamin B_6 in human nutrition. *Journal of the American Medical Association,* 1939, *112*(23), 2414-5.

Spittle, C. R. Atherosclerosis and vitamin C. *The Lancet,* 1971, *1*(7737), 1280-1.

Spittle, C. R. Atherosclerosis and vitamin C. *The Lancet,* 1972, *1*(7754), 798.

Sporn, M. B., Dunlop, N. M., Newton, D. L. and Smith, J. M. Prevention of chemical carcinogenesis by vitamin A and its synthetic analogs (retinoids), Federation Proceedings, 1976, *35,* 1332-1338.

Stamler, J. Comprehensive treatment of essential hypertensive disease. *Monograph on Hypertension.* West Point, Pennsylvania: Merck, Sharp and Dohme, 1970 (13).

Stamler, J. Why and how to prevent atherosclerotic diseases. *Giornale Italiana di Cardiologia,* 1974, *4,* 95-112.

Stamler, J. Diet-related risk factors for human atherosclerosis: Hyperlipidemia, hypertension, hyperglycemia, current status. *Advances in Experimental Medicine and Biology,* 1975, *60,* 125-158.

Stare, J. Proper eating has become a science. Journal of the *American Geriatrics Society,* 1962, *10*(9), 737-42.

Stare, J. (Ed.), *Athersclerosis.* New York: Medcom, Inc., 1974.

Stare, F. J. and McWilliams, M. *Living Nutrition.* New York: John Wiley and Sons, Inc., 1973, 338-339.

Steiner, D. F., Kemmler, W., Clark, J. L., Oyer, P. E. and Rubenstein, A. H. The biosynthesis of insulin. R. O. Greep and E. B. Astwood (Eds.) *Handbook of Physiology, Section 7 Endocrinology VI. Endocrine Pancreas.* Washington, D.C.: American Physiology Society, 1972, 175-198.

Steinkamp, R. C., Cohen, N. L. and Walsh, H. E. The San Mateo nutrition study. Resurvey of an aging population — 14-year follow-up. *Journal of the American Dietetic Association,* 1965, *46*(2), 103-10.

Strachan, R. W. and Henderson, J. G. Dementia and folate deficiency. *Quarterly Journal of Medicine,* 1967, *36,* 189.

Strehler, B. L., Hendley, D. D. and Hirsch, G. P. Evidence on a codon restriction hypothesis of cellular differentiation: Multiplicity of mammalian Leucyl-sRNA-specific synthetases and tissue-specific deficiency in an Alanyl-sRNA synthetase. *Proceedings of the National Academy of Science,* United States, 1967, *57,* 1751.

Strode, J. E. The large intestine as a geriatric problem. *Geriatrics,* 1968, 23(7), 102-12.

Stuart, R. B. Behavioral control of overeating. *Behavior Research and Therapy (Oxford),* 1967, *5,* 357-65.

Stuart, R. B. and Davis, B. *Slim Chance in a Fat World: Behavioral Control of Obesity.* Champaign, Illinois: Research Press, 1971.

Stunkard, A. New therapies for the eating disorders. *Archives of General Psychiatry,* 1972, *26*(5), 391-8.

Stunkard, A., and McLaren-Hume, M. The results of treatment for obesity. *Archives of Internal Medicine,* 1959, *103,* 79-85.

Sutherland, E. W. On the biological role of cyclic AMP. *Journal American Medical Association,* 1970, *214,* 1281.

Tanner, J. M. Growing up. *Scientific American,* 1973, *229*(3) 16-25.

Tanner, O. *Stress.* New York: Time-Life Books, 1976, 134.

Tappel, A. L. Vitamin E. *Nutrition Today,* 1973, *8*(4), 4-12.

Taylor, G. Vitamins and the elderly. *The Lancet,* 1974, *1*(7864), 1003.

Taylor, G. Diet and western disease. *The Lancet,* 1975, *1*(7907), 644.

Taylor, T. G. Nutrition and the elderly. *Modern Geriatrics,* 1973a, *3*(7), 350-1.

Taylor, T. G. Adding protein, subtracting carbohydrates equals better nutrition. *Geriatrics,* 1973b, *28*(11), 154-6.

Ten State Survey, 1968-1970. U.S. Department of Health Education and Welfare. State Nutrition Survey, 1968-70. Atlanta, Georgia: Center for Disease Control, H.E.W. Dept. (DHEW Publ.), V-1-5, HE 20.2302: N95/968-970, 1972.

Theuer, R. C. Nutrition and old age: A review. *Journal of Dairy Science,* 1971, *54*(5), 627-33.

Tobin, J. D., Sherwin, R. S., Liljenquist, J. E., Insel, P. A. and Andres, R. Insulin sensitivity and kinetics in men. In D. F. Chebotgrev, V. V. Frolkis, and A. Y. Mints (Eds.), *Proceedings of the 9th International Congress of Gerontology,* Kiev, U.S.S.R.: The Congress, 1972, 155.

Todhunder, N. E. Lifestyle and nutrient intake in the elderly. In M. Winick (Ed.), *Nutrition and Aging.* New York: John Wiley and Sons, 1976, 119-127.

Tomkin, G. H. Malabsorption of vitamin B_{12} in diabetic patients, with phenformin: A comparison with metformin. *British Medical Journal,* 1973, *3,* 673-675.

Trowell, H. C. *Non-infective Disease in Africa.* London: Edward Arnold, 1960, 217-222.

Trowell, H. C. Ischemic heart disease and dietary fibre. *American Journal of Clinical Nutrition,* 1972, *25,* 926.

Trowell, H. Definition of dietary fiber and hypothesis that it is a protective factor in certain diseases. *American Journal Clinical Nutrition,* 1976, *29,* 417.

Truswell, S. A. Food fiber and blood lipids. *Nutrition Reviews,* 1977, *35*(3), 51-54.

Tsai, A. C., Elia, J., Kelley, J. J., Linn, R.S.C. and Robson, R.R.K. Influence of certain dietary fibers on serum and tissue cholesterol levels in rats. *Journal of Nutrition,* 1976, *106,* 118.

Tunbridge, R. E. Nutrition and old age. *Practitioner,* 1961, *187,* (1118), 169-72.

Turner, J. S. *The Chemical Feast: Report on the Food and Drug Administration.* New York: Grossman, 1970.

Turpeinen, O., Miettinen, M. and Karvonen, M. J. *et al.* Dietary prevention of coronary heart disease. *American Journal of Clinical Nutrition,* 1968, *21,* 255.

Unger, R. Glucagon physiology and pathophysiology. *New England Journal of Medicine,* 1971, *285,* 443-449.

U.S. Congress Senate Special Committee on Aging. *Drugs in Nursing Homes: Issues, High Costs and Kickbacks.* Washington, D.C.: U.S. Government Printing Office, 1975.

U.S. Department of Health, Education and Welfare. Ten-state

nutrition survey. Atlanta, Georgia: Center for Disease Control, H.E.W. Dept. (DHEW Pub.) V-1-5, HE 20.2302:N95/968-70, 1972.

U.S. Department of Health Education and Welfare. Haynes Study. First health and nutrition examination survey, Public Number 74-1291-1, 1974, 7-18.

U.S. Government Printing Office. *Final Report of the White House Conference on Food, Nutrition and Health.* Washington, D.C.: U.S. Government Printing Office, 1970.

Vander, J. A., Sherman, J. H. and Luciano, D. C. Regulation of water and electrolyte balance. *Human Physiology: The Mechanisms of Body Function.* New York: McGraw-Hill Company, 1975, 319-354.

Vitale, J. J. Possible role of nutrients in neoplasia. *Cancer Research,* 1975, *35,* 3320-3325.

Wacker, E. C. Magnesium metabolism. *Journal American Dietetics Association,* 1964, *44,* 362.

Wacker, W. E. C. and Parisi, A. F. Magnesium metabolism. *New England Journal of Medicine,* 1968, *278,* 658, 712, 772.

Walford, R. L. *The Immunologic Theory of Aging.* Copenhagen: Muskgaard, 1969.

Walford, R., Liu, R. K. Gerbase-Delema, M., Mathies, M. and Smith, G. S. Long term dietary restriction and immune function in mice. *Mechanisms of Aging and Development,* 1973, *2,* 447-454.

Walker, A. R. P. Dietary fiber and the pattern of diseases. *Annals of Internal Medicine,* 1974, *80,* 663.

Walker, W. J. Changing United States life-style and declining vascular mortality: Cause or coincidence. *New England Journal of Medicine,* 1977, *297*(3), 163-165.

Watkin, D. M. Nutrition and aging. In B. H. Beaton and E. W. McHenry (Eds.), *Nutrition: A Comprehensive Treatise.* New York: Academic Press, 1966, 147-85.

Watkin, D. M. Nutritional problems today in the elderly in the United States. In A. N. Exton-Smith, and D. L. Scott (Eds.), *Vitamins in the Elderly.* Bristol: Wright & Sons, 1968, 66-77.

Watkin, D. M. Nutrition for the aging and the aged. In R. S. Goodhart and N. E. Shils (Eds.), *Modern Nutrition in*

Health and Disease. Philadelphia: Lea & Febiger, 1973, 681-710.

Weg, R. B. Drug interaction with the changing physiology of the aged: Practice and potential. In R. Davis (Ed.), *Drugs and the Elderly.* Los Angeles: Andrus Gerontology Center, 1973, 71-91.

Weg, R. B. Changing physiology of aging: Normal and pathological. In D. S. Woodruff and J. E. Birren (Eds.), *Aging: Scientific Perspectives and Social Issues.* New York: D. Van Nostrand Company, 1975, 229-256.

Weg, R. B. Changing physiology of aging. In R. H. Davis (Ed.), *Aging: Prospects and Issues.* Los Angeles: Andrus Gerontology Center, 1976, 58-69.

Weininger, J. and Briggs, G. M. Nutrition update. *Journal of Nutrition Education,* 1976, *8*(4), 172-175.

Werner, I. and Hambraeus, L. The digestive capacity of elderly people. In L. A. Carlson (Ed.), *Nutrition in Old Age.* Uppsala: Swedish Nutrition Foundation, 1972, 65-60.

West, M. and Kalbfleisch, J. M. Diabetes in Central America. *Diabetes,* 1970, *19*(9), 656-63.

Wester, P. O. Zinc during diuretic treatments. *The Lancet,* 1975, *1*,(7906), 578.

Whanger, A. D. Vitamins and vigor at 65 plus. *Postgraduate Medicine,* 1973, *53*(2), 167-72.

Whedon, G. D. Symposium comment. In U. S. Barzel (Ed.), *Osteoporosis.* New York: Grune and Stratton, 1970, 266-272.

White, P., Dahlquist, A., Pilnik, W. and Trowell, H. Summary of food and fibre symposium. *Nutrition* Reviews, 1977, *35*(3), 71-72.

Whitney E. and Hamilton, M. *Understanding Nutrition.* Los Angeles: West Publishing Company, 1977, 429-441.

Widdowson, E. M. and Dauncey, M. J. Obesity (ch 3 17-23) in *Present Knowledge in Nutrition.* Washington, D.C.: Nutrition Foundation, Inc., 1976.

Williams, R. J. We abnormal normals. *Nutrition Today,* 1967, *2,* 19-23.

Willis, G. C. An experimental study of intimal ground substance in atherosclerosis. *Canadian Medical Association Journal,* 1953, *69,* 17-22.

Wilson, C. W. M. The common cold and vitamin C: Prophylactic, therpeutic, metabolic and functional aspects. *Acta Vitaminologica et Enzymologica,* 1974, *28*(1/4), 96-98.

Winick, M. Malnutrition and brain development. *Journal of Pediatrics,* 1969, *74, 667.*

Witting, L. A. Vitamin E as a food additive. *Journal of the American Oil Chemists' Society (Chicago),* 1975, *52*(2), 64-8.

World Health Organization Technical Reports, (WHO Scientific Group) Nutritional anemias, 1968, (405).

World Health Organization Technical Reports, (FAO/WHO Expert Group), Requirements of ascorbic acid, Vitamin D, B_{12}, folate and iron. 1970, (452).

Wurtman, R. J. and Fernstrom, J. D. Effects of the diet on brain neurotransmitters. *Nutrition Reviews,* 1974, *32*(7), 193-200.

Wurtman, R. J., Rose, C. M., Chou, C. and Larin, F. Daily rhythms in the concentrations of various amino acids in human plasma. *New England Journal of Medicine,* 1968, 279, 171-175.

Wynder, E. L., Bross, J. J. A study of etological factors in cancer of the esophagus. *Cancer,* 1961, *14,* 389-413.

Wynder, E. L., Kojitani, T., Ishikawa, S., Dodo, H. and Takano, A. Environmental factors of cancer of the colon and rectum, II. Japanese epidemiological data. *Cancer,* 1969, *23*(5), 1210-20.

Yiengst, J. and Shock, W. Effect of oral administration of vitamin A on plasma levels of vitamin A and carotene in aged males. *Journal of Gerontology,* 1949, *4*(3) 205-11.

Young, V. R., Haververg, L. N., Bilmaze, S. C. and Munro, H. N. Potential use of three methylhistidine excretion as an index of progressive reduction in muscle protein catabolism during starvation. *Metabolism,* 1973a, *22,* 1429.

Young, V. R., Taylor, Y. S. M., Rand, W. M. and Scrimshaw, N. S. Protein requirements of man: Efficiency of egg protein maintenance and submaintenance levels in young men. *Journal of Nutrition,* 1973b, *103,* 1164.

Young, V. R., Steffee, W. P., Pencharz, P. B., Winterer, J. C.

and Scrimshaw, N. S. Total human body protein synthesis in relation to protein requirements at various ages. *Nature,* 1975, *253*(5488, 192-4.

Young, V. R. Protein metabolism and need in elderly people. In M. Rockstein and M. L. Sussman (Eds.), *Nutrition, Longevity and Aging.* New York: Academic Press, Inc., 1967a, 67-102.

Young, V. R., Perera, W. D., Winterer, J. C. and Scrimshaw, N. W. Protein and amino acid requirements of the elderly. In M. Winick (Ed.), *Nutrition and Aging.* New York: John Wiley and Sons, 1976b.

Yudkin, J. and Szanto, S. Relationship between sucrose intake, plasma insulin, and platelet adhesiveness in men with and without occlusive atherosclerosis. *Proceedings of the Nutrition Society,* 1970, *29,* 2A.

Yudkin, J., Edleman, J. and Hough, L. (Eds.), Sugar: *Chemical, Biological and Nutritional Aspects of Sucrose.* London: Butterworths, 1971.

Yudkin, J. Sugar and disease. *Nature,* 1972, 239(5369), 197-99.

200

Appendix 3

RDA VALUES
NUTRIENT CONTENT OF FOODS

Sources and Amounts of
Selected Nutrients in Common Foods

Acknowledgement:

Food sources of the selected nutrients on the following pages were chosen from LAUREL'S KITCHEN, published 1976 by Nilgiri Press, Box 477, Petaluma, California 94952.

In describing the energy requirements of adults, the FAO Committee on Calorie Requirements[1] adopted the concept of a *reference man and a reference woman.* This was continued, with changes in definition, by subsequent committees[2] in the belief that it was a useful approach to the estimation of energy requirements of population groups. The definitions of the reference man and woman as used in Table 1 are as follows:

> *The moderately active reference man* is between 20 and 40 years of age and weighs 65 kg. He is healthy — that is, free from disease and physically fit for active work. On each working day he is employed for 8 hours in an occupation that usually involves moderate activity. When not at work, he spends 8 hours in bed, 4-6 hours sitting or moving around in only very light activities and 2 hours in walking, in active recreation, or in household duties. Moderately active healthy men with these characteristics require an average of 3000 kcal/day (12.5 MJ/day) — that is to say, 46 kcal per kilogram per day (0.19 MJ/kg/day).

> *The moderately active reference woman* is between 20 and 40 years of age and weighs 55 kg. She is healthy — that is, free from disease and physically fit for active work. On each working day she is engaged for 8 hours in general household work, light industrial work, or other moderately active work. When not at work she spends 8 hours in bed, 4-6 hours in sedentary or very light activities and 2 hours in walking or more active recreation or duties. Moderately active healthy women with these characteristics require an average of 2200 kcal/day (9.2 MJ/day) — that is to say, 40 kcal/kg/day (0.17 MJ/kg/day).

[1] From: Nutrition in Preventive Medicine, Beaton, G. H. & Bengoa, J. M., World Health Organization, Geneva, 1976, p459, 460.

[2] WHO Technical Report Series, No. 522, 1973 (Report of a joint FAO/WHO *Ad HOC* Expert Committee on Energy and Protein Requirements)

RECOMMENDED DAILY DIETARY ALLOWANCES (RDA), U.S.A.

Food and Nutrition Board, National Research Council (Revised 1974)*

	Age years	Weight kg	lbs	Height cm	in	Energy kcal	Protein g	Vit. A[a] RE[h]	IU	Vit. D IU	Vit. E[e] IU	Vit. C mg
Infants	0 – ½	6	14	60	24	kgX117	kgX2.2	420	1400	400	4	35
	½ – 1	9	20	71	28	kgX108	kgX2.0	400	2000	400	5	35
Children	1 – 3	13	28	86	34	1300	23	400	2000	400	7	40
	4 – 6	20	44	110	44	1800	30	500	2500	400	9	40
	7 – 10	30	66	135	54	2400	36	700	3300	400	10	40
Men	11 – 14	44	97	158	63	2800	44	1000	5000	400	12	45
	15 – 18	61	134	172	69	3000	54	1000	5000	400	15	45
	19 – 22	67	147	172	69	3000	54	1000	5000	400	15	45
	23 – 50	70	154	172	69	2700	56	1000	5000		15	45
	51 +	70	154	172	69	2400	56	1000	5000		15	45
Women	11 – 14	44	97	155	62	2400	44	800	4000	400	12	45
	15 – 18	54	119	162	65	2100	48	800	4000	400	12	45
	19 – 22	58	128	162	65	2100	46	800	4000	400	12	45
	23 – 50	58	128	162	65	2000	46	800	4000		12	45
	51 +	58	128	162	65	1800	46	800	4000		12	45
Pregnant[g]						+300	+30	1000	5000	400	15	60
Lactating[h]						+500	+20	1200	6000	400	15	80

RECOMMENDED INTAKES OF NUTRIENTS, FAO/WHO†

	Age	kg	lbs	Energy kcal	Protein	Vit. A	Vit. D	Vit. C
Children	under 1	7.3	16	820	[i]14	[j]300 µg	[k]10.0 µg	20
	1 – 3	13.4	29	1360	[i]16	[j]250	[k]10.0	20
	4 – 6	20.2	44	1830	[i]20	[j]300	[k]10.0	20
	7 – 9	28.1	62	2190	[i]25	[j]400	[k]2.5	20
Men	10 – 12	36.9	81	2600	[i]30	[j]575	[k]2.5	20
	13 – 15	51.3	113	2900	[i]37	[j]725	[k]2.5	30
	16 – 19	62.9	138	3070	[i]38	[j]750	[k]2.5	30
	adult	65.0	143	3000	[i]37	[j]750	[k]2.5	30
Women	10 – 12	38.0	83	2350	[i]29	[j]575	[k]2.5	20
	13 – 15	49.9	110	2490	[i]31	[j]725	[k]2.5	30
	16 – 19	54.4	119	2310	[i]30	[j]750	[k]2.5	30
	adult	55.0	121	2200	[i]29	[j]750	[k]2.5	30
Pregnant[g]				+350	[i]38	[j]750	[k]10.0	30
Lactating[h]				+550	[i]46	[j]1200	[k]10.0	30

*Allowances are intended to provide for individual variations among most normal persons as they live in the U.S. under usual environmental stresses. If the RDA are met from a variety of common foods, the diet will also provide other nutrients for which human requirements are not so well defined. (See text.)

†U.N. recommendations, 1961-1972.

[a]Assumed to be as retinol in milk during first 6 months of life. All later intakes are assumed to be half as retinol and half as beta-carotene when calculated from international units; as retinol equivalents, three fourths are as retinol and one fourth as beta-carotene.

[b]Retinol equivalents. One retinol equivalent = 1 µg of retinol or 6 µg of beta-carotene.

[c]Total vitamin E activity, estimated to be 80% as alpha-tocopherol and 20% other tocopherols.

[d]Allowances refer to dietary sources; pure folacin may be effective in doses less than one-fourth the RDA.

Folacin[d] μg	Niacin[e] mg	Riboflavin mg	Thiamin mg	Vit. B-6 mg	Vit. B-12 μg	Calcium mg	Phos-phorus mg	Iodine μg	Iron mg	Mag. nesium mg	Zinc mg
50	5	0.4	0.3	0.3	0.3	360	240	35	10	60	3
50	8	0.6	0.5	0.4	0.3	540	400	45	15	70	5
100	9	0.8	0.7	0.6	1.0	800	800	60	15	150	10
200	12	1.1	0.9	0.9	1.5	800	800	80	10	200	10
300	16	1.2	1.2	1.2	2.0	800	800	110	10	250	10
400	18	1.5	1.4	1.6	3.0	1200	1200	130	18	350	15
400	20	1.8	1.5	2.0	3.0	1200	1200	150	18	400	15
400	20	1.8	1.5	2.0	3.0	800	800	140	10	350	15
400	18	1.6	1.4	2.0	3.0	800	800	130	10	350	15
400	16	1.5	1.2	2.0	3.0	800	800	110	10	350	15
400	16	1.3	1.2	1.6	3.0	1200	1200	115	18	300	15
400	14	1.4	1.1	2.0	3.0	1200	1200	115	18	300	15
400	14	1.4	1.1	2.0	3.0	800	800	100	18	300	15
400	13	1.2	1.0	2.0	3.0	800	800	100	18	300	15
400	12	1.1	1.0	2.0	3.0	800	800	80	10	300	15
800	+2	+0.3	+0.3	2.5	4.0	1200	1200	125	18+	450	20
600	+4	+0.5	+0.3	2.5	4.0	1200	1200	150	18	450	25

Folacin μg	Niacin mg	Riboflavin mg	Thiamin mg	Vit. B-12 μg	Calcium mg	Iron mg
60	5.4	0.5	0.3	0.3	500–600	[l]5–10
100	9.0	0.8	0.5	0.9	400–500	[l]5–10
100	12.1	1.1	0.7	1.5	400–500	[l]5–10
100	14.5	1.3	0.9	1.5	400–500	[l]5–10
100	17.2	1.6	1.0	2.0	600–700	[l]5–10
200	19.1	1.7	1.2	2.0	600–700	[l]9–18
200	20.3	1.8	1.2	2.0	500–600	[l]5–9
200	19.8	1.8	1.2	2.0	400–500	[l]5–9
100	15.5	1.4	0.9	2.0	600–700	[l]5–10
200	16.4	1.5	1.0	2.0	600–700	[l]12–24
200	15.2	1.4	0.9	2.0	500–600	[l]14–28
200	14.5	1.3	0.9	2.0	400–500	[l]14–28
400	+2.3	+0.2	+0.1	3.0	1000–1200	m
300	+3.7	+0.4	+0.2	2.5	1000–1200	m

[e]Although allowances are expressed as niacin, an average of 1 mg of niacin will also be contributed by every 60 mg of dietary tryptophan. (See p. 408)

[f]This increased requirement cannot be met by ordinary diets; the Food and Nutrition Board recommends a supplementary source of iron.

[g]Latter half of pregnancy.

[h]First six months.

[i]As egg or milk protein ("balanced" or highly utilizable protein; see text).

[j]As micrograms of retinol (1965 recommendation); 0.3 μg of retinol ≅ 1 IU.

[k]As micrograms of cholecalciferol; 10 μg of calciferol ≅ 400 IU.

[l]Lower value should be used when more than 25% of the diet's calories come from animal foods; the higher value applies when animal foods supply less than 10% of the calories.

[m]Supplementation is recommended when iron stores are depleted at the beginning of pregnancy; if iron status is satisfactory, the regular recommended intake applies.

THE U.S. RDA

"U.S. Recommended Daily Allowances" — Food and Drug Administration standards for nutrition labeling of foods,* based on the 1968 RDA.

	Adults and children over 4	Infants and children under 4
Protein	65 grams	28 grams
Vitamin A	5000 IU	2500 IU
Vitamin C	60 milligrams	40 milligrams
Thiamin	1.5 milligrams	0.7 milligrams
Riboflavin	1.7 milligrams	0.8 milligrams
Niacin	20 milligrams	9 milligrams
Calcium	1 gram	0.8 grams
Iron	18 milligrams	10 milligrams
Vitamin D	400 IU	400 IU
Vitamin E	30 IU	10 IU
Vitamin B-6	2 milligrams	0.7 milligrams
Folacin	0.4 milligrams	0.2 milligrams
Vitamin B-12	6 micrograms	3 micrograms
Phosphorus	1 gram	0.8 grams
Iodine	150 micrograms	70 micrograms
Magnesium	400 milligrams	200 milligrams
Zinc	15 milligrams	8 milligrams
Copper	2 milligrams	1 milligrams
Biotin	0.3 milligrams	0.15 milligrams
Pantothenic acid	10 milligrams	5 milligrams

*Including foods that are also vitamin—mineral supplements. (Labels for nonfood vitamin—mineral supplements follow a slightly different format.) No dietary supplements will give you more than 150 percent of the U.S. RDA for any nutrient; larger quantities will be sold as drugs.

PROTEIN AND CALORIE CONTENT OF PROTEIN SOURCE FOODS.

	% Protein in edible portion	Calories per gram of protein	Limiting amino acids (% of ideal pattern)‡
DAIRY PRODUCTS & EGGS			
Nonfat dry milk	35.9	10	*
Whole dry milk	26.4	19	*
Cheddar cheese, ripened	25.0	16	*
Cottage cheese, uncreamed	17.0	5	*
creamed	13.6	8	*
Egg, whole (hen's)	12.9	13	*
Egg white	10.9	5	*
Cream cheese	8.0	47	T 86
Skim milk or buttermilk	3.6	10	*
Whole milk (cow's)	3.5	19	*
Yogurt, low-fat	3.4	15	*
Goat's milk	3.2	21	M†
Whey, fluid	0.9	29	*
GRAINS (RAW)			
Oatmeal	14.2	27	L 73
Wheat: hard red spring	14.0	24	L 56
white bread flour			
(80% extraction)	12.0	30	L 41
gluten	88.9	4	L 28, T 95
germ	26.6	14	*
bran	16.0	13	L 85
Triticale	14.0	†	L 60, T†, M†
Rye, whole-meal	12.1	28	L 67, T 69
Buckwheat	11.7	29	L 75
Bulgur wheat (parboiled)	11.2	32	L 51
Sorghum	11.0	30	L 40, T 95
Millet	9.9	33	L 67
Barley, pot	9.6	36	L 68
Cornmeal, whole-ground	9.2	39	L 53, T 57
Rice, brown	7.5	48	L 75
parboiled, "converted"	7.4	50	L 69
polished (white)	6.7	54	L 71

*No limiting amino acids
†Values not available
‡T=tryptophan, L=lysine, M=total methionine and cystine

PROTEIN & CALORIE CONTENT OF PROTEIN SOURCE FOODS (Continued)

	% Protein in edible portion	Calories per gram of protein	Limiting amino acids (% of ideal pattern)‡
LEGUMES (RAW)			
Soybeans	34.1	12	M 99
fermented (tempeh)	16.9	10	*
cake or curd (tofu)	7.8	9	*
Soy milk	3.4	10	*
Peanuts	26.0	22	L 70, M 92, T 96
Fava beans (broad beans)	25.1	13	M 58, T 81
Lentils	24.7	14	M 65, T 90
Mung beans	24.2	14	M 47, T 75
Peas	24.1	14	M 77, T 84
Black-eyed peas	22.8	15	M 86
Common (red,white,pinto,black)	22.5	15	M 73, T 95
Garbanzos (chickpeas)	20.5	18	T 81, M 85
Limas	20.4	17	T 75, M 86
NUTS & SEEDS			
Pumpkin seeds	29.0	19	L 76, M†
Sunflower seeds	24.0	23	L 71
Walnuts, black	20.5	31	*
Pistachios	19.3	31	T 95, L 96
Sesame seeds	18.6	30	L 54
Almonds	18.6	32	L 44, T 80
Cashews	17.2	33	L 91
Cocoa (high-fat)	16.8	18	L 97, M†
Walnuts (English or Persian)	14.8	44	L 30, T 95
Brazil nuts	14.3	46	L 55, T 90
Filberts (hazelnuts)	12.6	50	M 47, L 58
Pecans	9.2	75	L 89
Coconut (dried kernel)	7.2	92	L 69
Carob flour	4.5	40	T 57
VEGETABLES (RAW) *Immature seeds*			
Limas, green	8.4	15	M 83
Peas	6.3	13	M 72, T 95
Corn	3.5	27	T 59, L 73
Black-eyed peas (in pods)	3.3	13	T 95, M†

*No limiting amino acids
†values not available
‡T=tryptophan, L=lysine, M=total methionine and cystine

PROTEIN & CALORIE CONTENT OF PROTEIN SOURCE FOODS (Continued)

	% Protein in edible portion	Calories per gram of protein	Limiting amino acids (% of ideal pattern)‡
VEGETABLES RAW *Green leaves*			
Kale (without stems)	6.0	9	L 61, M 69
Brussels sprouts	4.9	9	M 58
Collards (without stems)	4.8	9	*
Pigweed and lambsquarters	4.2	10	*
Parsley	3.6	12	M†
Spinach	3.2	8	*
Turnip greens	3.0	9	M 69
Mustard greens	3.0	10	L 95, M 96
Swiss chard	2.4	10	L 78, T 96, M†
Beet greens	2.2	11	L 56, M 67, T 95
Watercress	2.2	9	M†
Other vegetables			
Red pepper (hot)	3.7	25	T 93, M†
Broccoli	3.6	9	M 96
Mushrooms	2.7	10	M 38, L 88, T 96
Cauliflower	2.7	10	M†
Asparagus	2.5	10	M 84, L 89
Okra	2.4	15	T 54, L 65, M 87
Beans, snap	1.9	17	M 82
Roots			
Potato	2.1	36	M 72, L 94
Yam	2.1	48	L 81
Sweet potato	1.7	67	L 67
Cassava	1.1	†	M 66, L 82
YEAST			
Brewer's	38.8	7	M 95
Torula	38.6	7	T 42
Active dry	36.9	8	T 87

*No limiting amino acids
†Values not available
‡T=tryptophan, L=lysine, M=total methionine and cystine
Adapted from Watt & Merrill 1964 (Ag. Handbook no. 8), FAO/WHO 1970, and Orr & Watt 1957

LINOLEIC ACID CONTENT OF FATS & OILS

Grams of linoleic acid in 1 tablespoon of fat or oil

	Linoleic acid	Calories
Corn oil	7	124
Cottonseed oil	7	124
Olive oil	1	124
Peanut oil	4	124
Safflower oil	10	124
Sesame oil	6	124
Soy oil	7	124
Better-Butter (made with safflower oil)	5	113
Better-Butter (made with soy oil)	3	113
Margarine (first ingred. liquid oil)	4	100
Margarine (first ingred. hydrogenated oil)	2	100
Butter	trace	100
Peanut butter (with vegetable shortening)	2	86
Mayonnaise (soy, cottonseed, & corn oils, & egg)	6	102

Adapted from Watt & Merrill 1964 (Ag. Handbook no. 8)

CHOLESTEROL CONTENT OF FOODS

Figures to the left of food names give cholesterol content in milligrams.

DAIRY FOODS & EGGS

35	butter, 1 tablespoon	18	part skim, 1 ounce
282	½ cup or 1 stick	25	Muenster, 1 ounce
22	whipped, 1 tablespoon	64	Neufchatel, 3-oz. pkg.
190	½ cup	27	Parmesan, 1 ounce
5	buttermilk, 1 cup	113	grated, 1 cup
	cheese:	28	Provolone, 1 ounce
25	American, 1-oz. slice	14	ricotta, 1 ounce
24	bleu, 1 ounce	9	part skim, 1 ounce
117	1 cup crumbled	35	Swiss, 1¼-oz. slice
25	brick, 1 ounce	26	processed, 1-oz. slice
26	Camembert, 1 ounce	6	cream: half & half, 1 tbsp.
35	1-1/3-oz. piece	105	1 cup
28	cheddar, 1 ounce	10	light, 1 tablespoon
112	1 cup shredded	158	1 cup
27	Colby, 1 ounce	20	heavy, 1 tablespoon
23	cottage: low-fat, 1 cup	316	1 cup
	packed	8	sour, 1 tablespoon
48	creamed, 1 cup	152	1 cup
	packed	252	egg, whole, 1 large
13	uncreamed, 1 cup	252	yolk, 1 large
	packed	53	ice cream, 1 cup
16	cream cheese, 1 tbsp.	85	rich, 1 cup
94	3-ounce package	26	ice milk, hardened, 1 cup
29	Edam, 1 ounce	36	soft-serve, 1 cup
28	Limburger, 1 ounce	0	margarine, vegetable fat
27	mozzarella, 1 ounce	34	milk, fluid: whole, 1 cup

22	low-fat (2%), 1 cup
5	nonfat, 1 cup
79	evaporated, 1 cup
105	condensed, 1 cup
	milk, dry instant:
31	whole, ¼ cup
3	skim, ¼ cup
10	mayonnaise, 1 tbsp.
154	1 cup
50	noodles, egg, 1 cup ckd.
36	white sauce: thin, 1 cup
33	medium, 1 cup
30	thick, 1 cup
17	yogurt, nonfat, 8 ounces
15	fruit-flavored, 8 oz.

MEAT

80	beef, 3 ounces, cooked
2000	brains, 3½ ounces, raw
48	caviar, 1 tablespoon
63	chicken, ½ breast, ckd.
47	1 drumstick, cooked
114	clams, 1 cup meat

125	crab, 1 cup cooked
34	frankfurter, 1 cooked
75	halibut, 1 fillet, cooked
335	heart, chicken, cooked
	1 cup diced
1125	kidneys, 1 cup slices, ckd.
83	lamb, 3 ounces, cooked
195	lard, 1 cup
372	liver, 3 ounces, cooked
123	lobster, 1 cup cubes, ckd.
106	mackerel, 1 fillet, cooked
120	oysters, 1 cup, raw
76	pork, 3 ounces, cooked
129	sardines, 1 can
192	shrimp, 1 cup, canned
102	tuna, 5½-ounce can
65	turkey: light, 3 oz., ckd.
86	dark, 3 ounces, ckd.
86	veal, 3 ounces, cooked

Source: Feeley et al. 1972

SOME COMMON CARBOHYDRATES & THEIR SOURCES

MONOSACCHARIDES (SINGLE SUGARS)

GLUCOSE: corn syrup, grape sugar, vegetables, honey
FRUCTOSE: honey, fruits, vegetables
GALACTOSE: produce of lactose after digestion

DISACCHARIDES (DOUBLE SUGARS)

SUCROSE (glucose + fructose):
    cane, beet, maple, sorghum sugars; fruits & vegetables
LACTOSE (galactose + glucose):
    milk
MALTOSE (glucose + glucose):
    sprouting grains, beer

POLYSACCHARIDES (CHAINS OF SIMPLE SINGLE SUGARS)

STARCH: grains, legumes, vegetables
GLYCOGEN: in liver & muscle for energy storage; not found in plant or dairy foods
CELLULOSE: plants (indigestible structural components)
PECTINS: ripe fruits (absorb water & form jel as in fruit jellies)

FIBER CONTENT OF SOME COMMON FOODS*

- Recent studies indicate a number of potential health benefits from adequate food fiber intake.
- Good sources of food fibers include fruits, vegetables, whole grains, nuts, legumes.
- Six grams of crude fiber daily is suggested for healthy individuals with no problems related to the intestinal tract. (See discussion)
- The average American does not include this amount of fiber in his dietary choices.
- This table will give a factual basis for comparing and choosing foods which will contribute to this dietary essential.

Food (3½ oz.)	Fiber (grams)	Food (3½ oz.)	Fiber (grams)
Apple	1.0	Mustard greens,	
Apricot, unckd.	0.6	frozen, ckd.	1.0
Artichokes, ckd.	2.4	Oatmeal, ckd.	0.2
Asparagus, spears, ckd.	0.7	Oranges, raw peeled	0.5
Avocado	1.5	Orange juice	0.1
Banana	0.5	Papaya	0.9
Beans, white or red, ckd.	1.5	Parsnips	2.0
Beans, Lima, immature, ckd.	1.8	Peaches, canned	0.4
Bean Sprouts, (Mung		Peaches, raw	0.6
bean) raw or ckd.	0.7	Peanuts, roasted w/skin	2.7
Beans, green, ckd.	1.0	Peanut butter	1.8
Beet green, ckd.	1.1	Peas, green, ckd.	2.0
Blackberries, raw	4.1	Pecans	2.3
Blueberries, raw	1.5	Pepper pods, hot	
Bran flakes (40% bran)	3.6	chili, canned	1.2
Bran muffins	1.8	Persimmons, raw	1.5
Brans, wheat	7.8	Pineapple, raw	0.4
Brazil nuts	3.1	Pineapple juice	0.1
Breads, American rye	0.4	Pistachio nuts	1.9
Breads, cracked wheat	0.5	Plums, raw	0.4
Breads, white	0.2	Popcorns	2.2
Breads, whole wheat	1.6	Potatoes, bkd.	0.6
Broccoli, spears, boiled	1.5	Potatoes, mashed	0.4
Buckwheat, whole grain	9.9	Prunes, dried, unckd.	1.6
Buckwheat, flour, dark	1.6	Prune juice	trace
Buckwheat, flour, light	0.5	Pumpkin, canned	1.3
Cabbage, raw or ckd.	0.8	Pumpkin & squash	
Carrot, raw or ckd.	1.0	seed, kernels, dry	1.9
Celery	0.6	Radishes	0.7
Corn, ckd.	0.7	Raisins, unckd.	0.9
Cornbread, whole-ground	0.5	Raspberries, red, raw	3.0
Dates, natural, dry	2.3	Rhubarb, ckd.	0.6
Figs, dried, unckd.	5.6	Rice, brown, ckd.	0.3
Grapefruit	0.2	Rice, white, ckd.	0.1
Grapes	0.6	Rice brans	11.5
Jicama (yambean) raw	0.7	Rice, puffed	0.6
Lentils, mature, ckd.	1.2	Sapodilla, raw	1.4
Lettuce	0.5	Sapote	1.9
Mushrooms, canned	0.6	Sauerkraut, canned	0.7

Food (3½ oz.)	Fiber (grams)	Food (3½ oz.)	Fiber (grams)
Seaweed, kelp, raw	6.8	Tomatoes, raw	0.5
Soybean, ckd.	1.6	Tomato juice	0.2
Spinach, raw or ckd.	0.6	Turnips, ckd.	0.9
Squash, summer,		Turnip greens, ckd.	0.7
raw or ckd.	0.6	Vegetables, frozen, mixed	1.2
Squash, winter, bkd.		Walnuts, English	2.1
Strawberries, raw	1.3	Watercress, raw	0.7
Sunflower seed		Watermelon	0.3
kernels, dry	3.8	Wheat cereals	
Sweet potatoes, bkd.	0.9	(flk. shrd.)	1.6
		Wheat, germ	2.5

*Note: Crude fiber content of foods is obtained in the laboratory by treating the item with acid, alkali and/or alcohol. In the body, the digestive treatment is not as drastic, so the actual fiber content of food eaten by humans may be two to three times the amounts given above.

USDA COMPOSITION OF FOODS, Handbook No. 8, Washington: U.S. Government Printing Office, 1976.

FAT SOLUBLE VITAMINS

Vitamin A

CAROTENE; PROVITAMIN A; RETINOL

SOURCES

Adult RDA is 4000-5000 IU

22000	sorrel, 1 cup cooked
19000	lambsquarters, 1 c. ckd.
15000	carrots, 1 cup cooked
13000	butternut squash, 1 cup baked
12000	dandelion greens, 1 cup cooked
9800	Hubbard squash, 1 cup baked
9200	sweet potato, ckd., 1 lg.
9200	cantaloupe, ½ melon
9100	turnip greens, 1 c. ckd.
9100	kale, 1 cup cooked
8100	mustard greens, 1 c. ckd.
7400	beet greens, 1 c. cooked
5300	bok choy, 1 c. cooked
5300	papaya, 1 medium
4600	persimmon, 1 medium
4500	broccoli, ckd., 1 stalk
4500	spinach, raw, 1 cup chopped
3300	red pepper, sweet, raw
2900	apricots, 2 to 3 medium
2300	nectarine, 1 medium
2200	acorn squash, ½ baked
1400	romaine lettuce, 4 leaves
1300	peach, 1 medium
1300	asparagus, 1 cup cooked
1200	butter lettuce, 8 large leaves
1100	tomato, raw, 1 medium
750	prunes, with juice, 5 ckd.
630	grapefruit, pink, ½
590	egg, 1 large
470	butter, 1 tablespoon
470	margarine, fortified, 1 tablespoon
370	cheddar cheese, 1 ounce
350	milk, whole, 1 cup

Vitamin D
FOOD SOURCES (IU)

100 whole milk, fortified,
     8 fluid ounces
100 skim milk, fortified,
     8 fluid ounces
 27 egg yolk, 1 large
 14 butter, 1 tablespoon
  4 cream, light
     2 tablespoons
Tr buttermilk, 8 fl. oz.

VITAMIN E CONTENT OF FOODS

Values next to food names give vitamin E activity in International Units (IU).
Adult RDA is 12-15 IU.

OILS
.1   coconut, 1 tablespoon
3.6 corn, 1 tablespoon
8.9 cottonseed, 1 tablespoon
1.1 olive, 1 tablespoon
6.0 palm, 1 tablespoon
3.2 peanut, 1 tablespoon
4.6 rapeseed, 1 tablespoon
8.5 safflower, 1 tablespoon
3.4 sesame, 1 tablespoon
3.4 soybean, 1 tablespoon
10.3 sunflower, 1 tablespoon
13.1 walnut, 1 tablespoon
28.3 wheat germ, 1 tablespoon

NUTS & SEEDS
6.1 almonds, 15
1.4 brazil nuts, 4 medium
.1   chestnuts, 2 large
.2   coconut, ¼ c. dry shredded
4.7 filberts (hazelnuts), 10
1.4 peanuts, 1 tablespoon
.3   pecans, 12 halves
3.5 sunflower seeds, 2 tbsp.
4.6 walnuts, 8 to 15 halves

GRAINS & GRAIN PRODUCTS
.7   barley, whole-grain, ¼ cup dry
Tr   bread: white, 1 slice
.1   whole meal, 1 slice
.3   whole meal, germ-
     enriched, 1 slice
1.5 cornmeal, yellow, 1 cup
.2   millet, ¼ cup dry
.8   oatmeal, ½ cup dry

1.1 rice: brown, 1/3 cup dry
.1   white, ¼ cup dry
1.7 rye, whole-grain, 1/3 c. dry
.4   spaghetti, ¼ lb. dry
.1   tortilla, corn, 1 dried
1.5 wheat, whole-grain, 1/3 c. dry
Tr   wheat flour, bleached,
     1 cup sifted
.4   unbleached, 1 c. sifted
Tr   wheat bran, ¼ cup
4.2 wheat germ, ¼ cup

LEGUMES, MATURE
1.6 peas, ½ cup dry

VEGETABLES
.2   artichoke, 1 medium
3.7 asparagus, 5 to 6 spears
Tr   beans, snap, 1 cup cut

6.6 beet greens, ½ pound
2.2 broccoli, 5½" stalk
2.3 brussels sprouts, 3 large
 .3 cabbage, 1 cup shredded
 .6 carrot, 1 medium
 .2 cauliflowerets, 1 cup
 .3 celery, 1 med. outer stalk
1.5 corn, 1 medium ear
 .3 cucumber, 1 small
4.5 leeks, 3 to 4
 .2 lettuce, 1 cup chopped
 .1 mushrooms, 3 large
 .2 okra, 1 cup slices
 .5 onions, 1 cup chopped
 .2 parsley, August, ¼ c. chopped
 .7   November, ¼ c. chopped
1.5 parsnip, ½ large
 .2 peas, 1 cup
10.9 spinach, ½ pound
9.7 sweet potato, 1 medium
 .5 tomato, 1 medium
7.5 turnip greens, ½ pound
 .2 watercress, 10 sprigs

FRUITS
1.8 apple, 1 medium

 .7 banana, 1 medium
8.6 blackberries, wild, 1 cup
1.5   cultivated, 1 cup
 .2 cherries, 10
 .6 grapefruit, ½ medium
 .2 melon, 1 cup diced
 .4 orange, 1 medium
1.2 pear, 1 medium
 .6 plum, 1 large
 .8 raspberries, 1 cup
 .5 strawberries, 1 cup

DAIRY PRODUCTS & EGGS
 .5 butter, 1 tablespoon
0   egg white, 1 large
 .6 egg yolk, 1 large
 .3 milk (3.5% fat), 1 cup

MISCELLANEOUS
2.2 chocolate, unsweetened,
         1 ounce
Tr   molasses, 1 tablespoon
0   yeast: brewer's, 1 tbsp.
Tr   torula, 1 tablespoon

There are several different tocopherols in foods. Each tocopherol has a different level of biological activity, but only the activity of alpha- and gamma-tocopherol has been precisely determined. All values given here include alpha-tocopherol content; gamma-tocopherol content has been included also wherever data were available, as for all the oils. The resulting alpha-tocopherol equivalent, measured in milligrams, has been multiplied by 1.5 to give International Units (IU). Values are adapted from Slover 1971 and Dicks 1965.

WATER SOLUBLE VITAMINS

Vitamin C

ASCORBIC ACID

SOURCES
Adult RDA is 45 mg

FRESH FRUITS
240 guava, medium
170 papaya, medium
120 orange juice, 1 cup
90 cantaloupe, ½ melon
88 strawberries, 1 cup
81 mango, medium
66 orange, medium

54 grapefruit, ½ medium
39 lemon, medium
31 red raspberries, 1 cup
30 blackberries, 1 cup
27 tangerine, medium
26 pineapple, 1 cup diced
20 blueberries, 1 cup
12 banana, medium

RAW VEGETABLES
150   red pepper, sweet, med.
 94   green pepper, medium
 42   cabbage, 1 cup chopped
 28   tomato, medium
 28   spinach, 1 cup chopped
 20   mung bean sprouts, 1 cup

COOKED VEGETABLES
160   broccoli, 1 stalk
140   brussels sprouts, 8
140   collard greens, 1 cup
110   sorrel, 1 cup
100   kale, 1 cup
 74   lambsquarters, 1 cup

71   kohlrabi, 1 cup diced
70   green pepper, medium
69   cauliflowerets, 1 cup
67   mustard greens, 1 cup
58   tomato, 1 cup
50   spinach, 1 cup
48   cabbage, 1 cup
44   rutabagas, 1 cup sliced
34   turnip, 1 cup diced
32   peas, 1 cup
32   okra, 1 cup slices
29   green lima beans, 1 cup
28   chard leaves, 1 cup
25   sweet potato, baked
22   potato, boiled

Niacin

NICOTINIC ACID; NICOTINAMIDE; NIACINAMIDE

SOURCES
Niacin equivalent in milligrams (niacin content in mg plus 1 mg of niacin/60 mg of tryptophan) Adult RDA is 13-18 mg

15.6 tofu, 4 ounce piece
11.5 soybeans, ½ cup dry
 8.5 rice polishings, ¼ cup
 8.0 cottage cheese, 1 cup
 7.3 bulgur wheat, ¾ cup dry
 7.2 peas, ½ cup dry
 6.0 collard greens, ½ lb. raw
 5.8 navy beans, ½ cup dry
 5.6 mung beans, ½ cup dry
 5.6 peas, fresh, 1 cup
 5.5 pinto beans, ½ cup dry
 5.5 kidney beans, ½ cup dry
 5.3 lentils, ½ cup dry
 4.9 black-eyed peas, ½ c. dry
 4.8 garbanzos, ½ cup dry
 4.8 lima beans, ½ cup dry
 4.8 wheat berries, 1/3 c. dry
 4.7 green limas, 1 cup raw
 4.5 buckwheat, 1/3 cup dry
 4.5 oatmeal, ¾ cup dry
 4.4 torula yeast, 1 tablespoon
 4.0 avocado, ½ medium
 4.0 peanuts, 2 tablespoons
 3.9 brewer's yeast, 1 tbsp.
 3.7 rice, brown, 1/3 cup dry
 3.4 peanut butter, 1 tbsp.

3.2 wheat bran, ¼ cup
3.2 kale, ¼ pound raw
3.0 egg, 1 large
3.0 mushrooms, raw, 3 large
3.0 mango, 1 medium
2.8 potato, raw, 1 cup diced
2.8 spinach, ½ pound raw
2.7 rye berries, 1/3 cup dry
2.6 dates, 10 medium
2.5 millet, ¼ cup dry
2.5 brussels sprouts, 8 raw
2.3 broccoli, raw, 1 stalk
2.1 wheat germ, ¼ cup
2.1 milk, 1 cup
2.0 sesame seeds, 2 tbsp.
2.0 sunflower seeds, 2 tbsp.
1.9 asparagus, raw,
         5 to 6 spears
1.6 cantaloupe, ½ melon
1.5 cheddar cheese, 1 ounce
1.4 summer squash, raw,
         1 cup diced
1.4 banana, large
1.4 guava, medium
1.2 cornmeal, unbolted,
         1/3 cup dry

FOLACIN CONTENT OF FOODS

Values next to food names give total folate in micrograms (μg).
Adult RDA is 400 μg.

LEGUMES, MATURE
125 garbanzos, ½ cup dry
122 kidney beans, ½ cup dry
102 lima beans, ½ cup dry
33 peas, ½ cup dry
132 white beans, ½ cup dry
236 soybeans, ½ cup dry
298 soy flour, 1 cup stirred

VEGETABLES
64 asparagus, 5 to 6 spears
40 beans: wax, 1 cup pieces
44   green, 1 cup pieces
93 beets, 2 medium
72 broccoli, 1 medium stalk
97 brussels sprouts, 3 large
69 cabbage, 1 cup shredded
15 carrot, 1 medium
31 cauliflowerets, 1 cup
5 celery, 1 med. outer stalk
18 corn, 1 medium ear
27 cucumber, 1 small
13 eggplant, 2 slices
20 endive, 1 cup cut
102 lettuce, romaine, 1 cup cut
16 mushrooms, 3 lrg. or 7 sm.
27 onion: Spanish,
      1 cup chopped
2   green, bulb,
      1 tbsp. chopped
14 pepper: green, 1 med. pod
38   red, 1 medium pod
21 potato, fresh, 1 medium
20   after storage, 1 medium
11 radishes, 10 medium
463 spinach, ½ pound
31 squash, winter, 3½ oz.
84 sweet potato, 1 medium
7 tomato, 1 medium
26 turnip, 1 cup diced

FRUITS
10 apple, 1 medium
4 apricots, ¼ c. dried halves
41 avocado, ½ medium
36 banana, 1 medium
9 blueberries, 1 cup
49 cantaloupe, 1 cup diced
6 cherries, 10
17 dates, 10 medium

3 figs, 2 small dried
10 grapes: blue, 1 cup
4   red, 1 cup
6 grape juice, 1 cup
15 grapefruit, white, ½ med.
13   pink, ½ medium
52   juice, 1 cup
5 lemon, 1 medium
3 lime, 1 medium
7 nectarine, 1 medium
60 orange, 1 medium
164 orange juice, fresh, 1 cup
3 peach, 1 medium
19 pear, 1 medium
16 pineapple, 1 cup diced
1 plum, 1 yellow
2 prunes, 5 large
1 raisins, ¼ cup
24 strawberries, 1 cup
18 tangerine, 1 medium
5 watermelon, 1 cup diced

GRAINS & GRAIN PRODUCTS
10 barley, pot, ¼ cup dry
11 bread: white, 1 slice
15   whole wheat, 1 slice
26   whole wheat, homemade,
      1 slice
7   rye, dark, 1 slice
30 cornmeal, 1 cup dry
31 flour: all-purpose, 1 c. sifted
80   whole wheat, 1 c. stirred
99   rye, dark, 1 cup
12 macaroni, ¼ pound dry
34 oatmeal, quick, ¾ cup dry
37 rice, long-grain, ¼ c. dry
15 spaghetti, ¼ pound dry
28 wheat, cracked, 1/3 c. dry
17 wheat bran, ¼ cup
52 wheat germ, ¼ cup

NUTS
14 almonds, 15
19 cashews, 14 large
8 coconut, fresh, shredded,
      ¼ cup
10 filberts (Hazelnuts), 10
13 peanut butter, 1 tbsp.
10 peanuts, 1 tbsp. chopped

4   pecans, 12 halves
9   pistachios, 30
10   walnuts, 8 large halves

DAIRY PRODUCTS & EGGS
6   cheddar cheese, mild, 1 oz.
3   egg white, 1 large
50   egg yolk, hard-cooked, 1 lrg.
37   milk, whole, 1 cup
27   yogurt, 1 cup

MISCELLANEOUS
3   molasses, light, 1 tbsp.
286   yeast: active dry, 1 tbsp.
308   brewer's, 1 tablespoon
240   torula, 1 tablespoon

Adapted from Butterfield &
Calloway 1972, Hoppner et al.
1972, and Dong & Oace 1973.

Vitamin B-2
RIBOFLAVIN

SOURCES
Adult RDA is 1.1-1.6 mg

.61   cottage cheese, 1 cup
.51   low-fat milk, 1 cup
.44   yogurt, low-fat, 1 cup
.41   whole milk, 1 cup
.40   torula yeast, 1 tablespoon
.38   collard greens, 1 c. cooked
.36   broccoli, cooked, 1 stalk
.34   brewer's yeast, 1 tbsp.
.32   mushrooms, 1 cup cut
.29   camembert cheese,
            1-1/3 oz. wedge
.29   okra, 1 cup cooked
.27   butternut squash, 1 c. baked
.26   almond meal, ¼ cup
.26   asparagus, 1 cup cooked
.26   cheddar cheese, 2 ounces
.26   sorrel, 1 cup cooked
.25   spinach, 1 cup cooked
.23   avocado, ½ medium
.22   beet greens, 1 cup cooked
.22   brussels sprouts, 1 c. ckd.
.22   millet, ¼ cup dry
.20   wheat germ, ¼ cup
.19   chard, 1 cup cooked
.18   split peas, green, 1 c. ckd.
.18   pinto beans, 1 cup cooked

Vitamin B-1
THIAMIN

SOURCES
Adult RDA is 1.0-1.5 mg

1.2   brewer's yeast, 1 tbsp.
1.1   torula yeast, 1 tbsp.
.66   whole wheat flour, 1 cup
.56   rice bran, ¼ cup
.51   pinto beans, 1 cup cooked
.48   rice polishings, ¼ cup
.45   peas, fresh, 1 cup cooked
.44   wheat germ, ¼ c. toasted
.42   millet, ¼ cup dry
.38   soybeans, 1 cup cooked
.38   wheat berries, 1/3 cup dry
.36   piñon nuts, 1 ounce
.36   sunseeds, 2 tbsp.
.35   black beans, 1 cup cooked
.33   barley, ¼ cup dry
.31   rye berries, 1/3 cup dry
.31   lima beans, green, 1 c. ckd.
.30   split peas, green, 1 c. ckd.
.27   navy beans, 1 cup cooked
.25   spinach, 1 cup cooked
.24   orange, 1 large
.23   avocado, ½ medium
.23   asparagus, 1 cup cooked
.20   kidney beans, 1 c. cooked
.19   oatmeal, 1 cup cooked
.18   rice, brown, 1 cup cooked
.18   sesame seeds, 2 tbsp.
.18   yam, 1 cup cooked
.18   wheat bran, ¼ cup
.16   broccoli, cooked, 1 stalk
.16   bulgur wheat, 1/3 cup dry
.15   whole wheat bread, 2 slices

Vitamin B-6
PYRIDOXINE

SOURCES
Adult RDA is 2.0 mg

.8	rice bran, ¼ cup
.8	rice polishings, ¼ cup
.85	soybeans, ½ cup dry
.68	kale, ½ pound raw
.64	spinach, ½ pound raw
.61	banana, medium
.57	buckwheat flour, 1 cup
.57	navy beans, ½ cup dry
.57	lentils, ½ cup dry
.54	garbanzo beans, ½ cup dry
.52	lima beans, ½ cup dry
.50	pinto beans, ½ cup dry
.48	black-eyed peas, ½ c. dry
.46	avocado, ½ medium
.41	whole wheat flour, 1 cup
.38	potato, raw, 1 cup diced
.38	rye flour, dark, 1 cup
.35	raisins, 1 cup
.34	rice, brown, 1/3 cup dry
.30	broccoli, raw, 1 stalk
.30	asparagus, raw, 12 to 14 spears
.30	wheat germ, ¼ cup
.26	brussels sprouts, 8 raw
.24	torula yeast, 1 tablespoon
.24	lima beans, green, frozen, 1 cup
.24	beet greens, ½ pound raw
.23	cantaloupe, ½ melon
.23	green peas, 1 cup raw
.22	sunflower seeds, 2 tbsp.
.22	sweet potato, raw, 1 small
.21	cauliflowerets, 1 cup raw
.20	brewer's yeast, 1 tbsp.
.20	leeks, 3 to 4 raw

Vitamin B-12
COBALAMIN

SOURCES
Adult RDA is 3.0 μg

1.2	cottage cheese, ½ c. packed
1.0	milk, whole or skim, 1 cup
1.0	egg, large
.95	dried skim milk, regular ¼ cup
.54	buttermilk, 1 cup
.50	Swiss cheese, 1 ounce
.50	edam cheese, 1 ounce
.49	camembert cheese, 1-1/3 ounce wedge
.39	bleu cheese, 1 ounce
.28	cheddar cheese, 1 ounce
.28	brick cheese, 1 ounce
.28	mozzarella cheese, 1 ounce
.28	whey, fluid, 7 tbsp.
.27	yogurt, 1 cup
.06	cream cheese, 1 ounce
.04	cream, light, 1 tablespoon

MAJOR MINERALS

SOURCES OF CALCIUM
Adult RDA is 800 mg

Spinach, chard, sorrel, beet greens, lambsquarters, parsley, chocolate, rhubarb, and wheat bran are not included since their calcium is poorly utilized, due to the oxalic acid content.

400	skim milk powder, ¼ cup	220	edam cheese, 1 ounce
360	collard leaves, 1 c. ckd.	210	cheddar cheese, 1 ounce
350	low-fat milk, 1 cup	200	kale, 1 cup cooked
300	buttermilk, 1 cup	180	mustard greens, 1 c. ckd.
290	whole milk, 1 cup	160	broccoli, cooked, 1 stalk
280	blackstrap molasses, 2 tbsp.	150	okra, cooked, 1 cup slices
270	sesame seed meal, ¼ cup	150	tofu, 4 ounce piece
270	yogurt, 1 cup	150	dandelion greens, 1 c. ckd.
270	Parmesan cheese, ¼ cup grated	140	Masa Harina, 1 cup dry
		130	soybeans, 1 cup cooked
260	Swiss cheese, 1 ounce	120	tortillas, 2
250	bok choy, 1 cup cooked	120	carob flour, ¼ cup
230	cottage cheese, 1 cup	100	rutabagas, 1 cup cooked

Other sources of calcium which can be utilized by the body include chalk, limestone, granite, eggshell, sea shells, and hard water.

SOURCES OF PHOSPHORUS
Adult RDA is 800 mg

430	pinto beans, 1 cup cooked	220	yogurt, 1 cup
420	black beans, 1 cup cooked	210	green lima beans, 1 c. ckd.
370	cottage cheese, 1 cup	200	pumpkin seeds, 2 tbsp.
350	rice bran, ¼ cup	180	buckwheat, 1/3 cup dry
330	garbanzo beans, 1 c. ckd.	160	Swiss cheese, 1 ounce
320	soybeans, 1 cup cooked	160	peas, fresh, 1 cup cooked
320	Masa Harina, 1 cup dry	150	tofu, 4 ounce piece
300	rice polishings, ¼ cup	150	corn, 1 cup cooked
300	skim milk powder, ¼ cup	140	sesame seed meal, ¼ cup
290	lima beans, 1 cup cooked	140	almond meal, ¼ cup
280	wheat bran, ¼ cup	140	nutritional yeast, 1 tbsp.
280	navy beans, 1 cup cooked	140	cheddar cheese, 1 ounce
270	rye berries, 1/3 cup dry	110	broccoli, cooked, 1 stalk
260	wheat berries, 1/3 cup dry	100	collard greens, 1 c. ckd.
260	kidney beans, 1 cup cooked	60	kale, 1 cup cooked
230	milk, 1 cup	60	bok choy, 1 cup cooked
230	wheat germ, ¼ cup		

SOURCES OF POTASSIUM (in milligrams)

1200	butternut squash, 1 cup baked	600	prune juice, 1 cup
		590	parsnips, 1 cup cooked
1200	lima beans, dry, 1 c. ckd.	590	split peas, 1 cup cooked
1160	spinach, 1 cup cooked	580	blackstrap molasses, 1 tablespoon
1000	black beans, 1 cup cooked		
970	soybeans, 1 cup cooked	520	dates, 10 medium
940	pinto beans, 1 cup cooked	500	potato, cooked
790	navy beans, 1 cup cooked	500	orange juice, 1 cup
750	acorn squash, ½ baked	490	skim milk powder, ¼ c.
720	green lima beans, 1 c. ckd.	480	beet greens, 1 cup
710	papaya, medium	440	banana, medium
680	cantaloupe, ½ melon	430	low-fat milk, 1 cup
650	avocado, ½ medium	430	kohlrabi, 1 cup cooked
650	raisins, ½ cup	420	peas, fresh, 1 cup
630	kidney beans, 1 c. ckd.	420	brussels sprouts, 1 c. ckd.
600	chard, 1 cup cooked	410	nectarine, medium

MAGNESIUM CONTENT OF FOODS

Values next to food names give magnesium content in milligrams. Adult RDA is 300-350 mg.

LEGUMES, MATURE

173	beans: white, ½ cup dry
150	red, ½ cup dry
196	black-eyed peas, ½ cup dry
76	lentils, ½ cup dry
162	limas, ½ cup dry
278	soybeans, ½ cup dry
173	soybean flour, full-fat, 1 c.
133	tofu, 2½"x2¾"x1"

GRAINS & GRAIN PRODUCTS

21	barley, pearl, ¼ cup dry
72	whole-grain, ¼ cup dry
8	breads: french, 1 slice
10	rye, light, 1 slice
23	pumpernickel, dark, 1 sl.
6	white, 1 slice
22	whole wheat, 1 slice
149	buckwheat, whole, 1/3 c. dry
47	flour, light, 1 cup
129	cornmeal, bolted, 1 c. dry
65	degermed, 1 cup dry
25	macaroni, ckd. tender, 1 c.
94	millet, ¼ cup dry
50	oatmeal, 1 cup cooked
57	rice, brown, 1 cup cooked
16	rice, white, 1 cup cooked
64	rye flour, light, 1 cup
107	wheat berries, 1/3 cup dry
64	wheat bran, ¼ cup
69	wheat germ, ¼ cup
136	whole wheat flour, 1 cup
29	all-purpose, 1 cup

NUTS & SEEDS

41	almonds, 15
34	brazil nuts, 4 medium
75	cashews, 14 large
14	coconut, dried, ¼ cup
28	filberts (hazelnuts), 10
19	peanuts, 1 tbsp. chopped
28	peanut butter, 1 tablespoon
21	pecans, 12 halves
24	pistachios, 30
33	sesame seeds, whole, 2 tbsp.
7	sunflower seeds, 2 tbsp.
15	walnuts: black, 4 to 5 halves
10	English, 4 to 7 halves

VEGETABLES

20	asparagus, 5 to 6 spears
35	beans, snap, 1 cup pieces
27	beets, 2 medium
241	beet greens, ½ pound
24	broccoli, 1 medium stalk
44	brussels sprouts, 3 large
9	cabbage, 1 cup shredded
17	carrot, 1 medium
24	cauliflowerets, 1 cup
9	celery, 1 outer stalk
148	chard, Swiss, ½ pound
129	collards, ½ pound
26	corn, 1 medium ear
82	dandelion greens, ½ lb.
16	eggplant, ½ cup diced
42	kale, ¼ pound
6	lettuce, head, 1 c. chopped
13	mushrooms, 4 large
61	mustard greens, ½ lb.
20	onion, 1 cup chopped
32	parsnip, ½ large
51	peas, 1 cup
13	pepper, green, 1 medium
51	potato, 1 medium
200	spinach, ½ pound
21	squash, summer, 1 c. diced
50	sweet potato, 1 medium
17	tomato, 1 medium
26	turnips, 1 cup diced
132	turnip greens, ½ pound

FRUITS

13	apple, 1 medium
10	apple juice, bottled, 1 cup
13	apricots, 2 to 3 medium
51	avocado, ½ medium
39	banana, 1 medium
43	blackberries, 1 cup
26	cantaloupe, 1 cup diced
46	dates, 10 medium
10	figs, fresh, 2 large
21	dried, 2 small
17	grapefruit, ½ medium
30	grape juice, bottled, 1 cup
5	lemon juice, ¼ cup
36	mango, 1 medium
18	nectarine, 1 medium
14	orange, 1 medium
27	orange juice, fresh, 1 cup
10	peach, 1 medium
20	pineapple, 1 cup diced
6	plum, 1 large
20	prunes, 5 cooked
26	prune juice, bottled, 1 cup

13   raisins, ¼ cup
18   strawberries, 1 cup

DAIRY PRODUCTS & EGGS
13   cheese: cheddar, 1-oz. slice
2   Parmesan, 1 tbsp. grated
2   cream, light, 1 tbsp.
5   egg, whole, 1 large
3   white of large egg
3   yolk of large egg
19   ice cream, 1 cup
32   milk, cow's: whole, 1 cup
34   skim, 1 cup
34   buttermilk, 1 cup
43   dry skim, regular, ¼ c.
24   dry skim, instant, ¼ c.

MISCELLANEOUS
30   chocolate, sweet, 1 oz.
21   cocoa, dry, 1 tablespoon
5   coffee, instant dry, 1 tsp.
Tr   mayonnaise, 1 tbsp.
2   salad dressing, french
        1 tablespoon
6   salt, 1 teaspoon
11   yeast: active, 1 cake
18   brewer's, 1 tablespoon
13   torula, 1 tablespoon

Adapted from Watt & Merrill 1964 (Ag. Handbook no. 8)

TRACE MINERALS

IRON CONTENT

SOURCES
Adult RDA is 10-18 mg

10.5   prune juice, 1 cup
7.9   black beans, 1 cup cooked
6.9   garbanzo beans, 1 c. ckd.
6.1   pinto beans, 1 c. ckd.
5.1   navy beans, 1 c. ckd.
5.1   lima beans, dry, 1 c. ckd.
4.9   soybeans, 1 cup cooked
4.8   rice bran, ¼ cup
4.4   rice polishings, ¼ cup
4.3   lima beans, green, 1 c. ckd.
4.2   lentils, 1 cup cooked
4.0   spinach, 1 cup cooked
3.9   peach halves, dried, 5
3.9   millet, ¼ cup dry
3.4   sunchokes, 4 small
3.4   split peas, green, 1 c. ckd.
3.2   blackstrap molasses,
        1 tablespoon
2.9   peas, fresh, 1 cup
2.8   beet greens, 1 c. cooked
2.6   raisins, ½ cup
2.6   chard, 1 cup cooked

2.4   dates, 10 medium
2.4   sesame meal, ¼ cup
2.3   tofu, 4 ounce piece
2.2   tomato juice, 1 cup
2.1   wheat berries, 1/3 cup dry
2.1   butternut squash,
        1 cup baked
2.0   pumpkin seeds, 2 tbsp.
1.9   wheat bran, ¼ cup
1.9   wheat germ, ¼ cup
1.8   soybean milk, 1 cup
1.8   kale, 1 cup cooked
1.8   prunes, 5 cooked
1.7   acorn squash, ½ baked
1.7   brussels sprouts, 8 cooked
1.5   torula yeast, 1 tbsp.
1.5   strawberries, 1 cup
1.4   potato, cooked, large
1.4   oatmeal, 1 cup cooked

ZINC CONTENT OF FOODS

Values next to food names give zinc content in milligrams (mg).
Adult RDA is 15 mg.

LEGUMES, MATURE
1.8   beans, common, 1 c. ckd.
3.0   black-eyed peas, 1 c. ckd.
2.0   garbanzos, 1 cup ckd.
2.0   lentils, 1 cup cooked
1.7   limas, 1 cup cooked
0.3   peanuts, roasted, 1 tbsp.
0.5   peanut butter, 1 tbsp.
2.1   peas, green, 1 cup ckd.

GRAINS & GRAIN PRODUCTS
0.1   barley, whole, ¼ cup dry
0.4   bread: rye, 1 slice
0.2   white, 1 slice
0.5   whole wheat, 1 slice
1.3   buckwheat, whole
          1/3 cup dry
0.7   corn grits, 1 cup dry
2.1   cornmeal, bolted, 1 c. dry
0.2   crackers, graham, 2
0.1   saltines, 10
0.6   granola, 1 ounce
0.7   macaroni, 1 cup cooked
0.9   millet, whole, ¼ cup dry
1.2   oatmeal, 1 cup cooked
3.1   rice bran, 1 cup
1.2   rice, brown, 1 cup ckd.
0.6   rice, white parboiled,
          1 cup cooked
1.4   soy flour, 1 cup stirred
5.9   soy meal, 3½ ounces
1.0   soy protein, ¼ cup
      wheat berries:
2.3   hard, 1/3 cup dry
1.8   soft, 1/3 cup dry
1.5   white, 1/3 cup dry
1.8   durum, 1/3 cup dry
5.7   wheat bran, 1 cup
3.2   wheat germ, toasted,
          ¼ cup
      wheat flours:
2.9   whole, 1 cup stirred
0.8   all-purpose, 1 cup sftd.
0.9   bread flour, 1 cup sftd.
0.3   cake flour, 1 cup sftd.
1.2   wheat cereal, whole-meal,
          1 cup cooked

DAIRY PRODUCTS & EGGS
0.2   butter, 1 cup
0.01   1 tablespoon
0.5   cheese, cheddar, 1 slice
0.5   egg, whole, 1 large
0.5   yolk, 1 large
0.01   white, 1 large
0.6   ice cream, 1 cup
0.9   milk, fluid, 1 cup
1.9   canned, evaporated, 1 cup
3.1   dry, nonfat, 1 cup

VEGETABLES
0.4   beans, snap green,
          French-cut, 1 cup ckd.
0.3   cabbage, common,
          shredded, 1 cup raw
0.6   1 cup boiled, drained
0.3   carrot, raw, 1 medium
0.5   1 cup cooked, drained
0.7   corn, sweet yellow,
          1 cup boiled, drained
0.4   lettuce, 1/6 head
0.2   loose-leaf, 1 cup chpd.
0.6   onions, mature,
          1 cup chopped
0.3   young green,
              1 cup chopped
1.2   peas, green immature,
          1 cup boiled, drained
0.3   potato, 1 medium pared,
          boiled, drained
0.4   1 medium boiled in
              skin, drained, pared
0.5   spinach, raw,
          1 cup chopped
1.3   1 cup boiled, drained
0.2   tomato, raw, 1 medium
0.5   1 cup boiled
0.5   1 cup canned, w. liq.

FRUITS
0.08 apple, 1 medium
0.3   applesauce,
          unsweetened, 1 cup
0.3   banana, 1 medium
0.2   orange, 1 medium
0.2   orange juice, canned, 1 cup
0.05   fresh or frozen, 1 cup
0.2   peach, raw peeled, 1 medium
0.3   canned, 1 cup slices

MISCELLANEOUS

0.01	beverages, carbonated, 12-ounce bottle
0.3	12-ounce can
1.6	cocoa, powder, 1 ounce
0.3	1 tablespoon
0.05	coffee, 6 fluid ounces
0.5	margarine, 1 cup
0.03	1 tablespoon
0.4	oil, salad or cooking, 1 cup
0.1	sugar, white granulated, 1 cup
0.04	tea, 6 fluid ounces
0.8	yeast, active dry, 1 tbsp.
0.4	brewer's, 1 tablespoon
0.8	torula, 1 tablespoon

Sources: Murphy et al. 1975, Prasad 1966

"The end of all knowledge is action"
Thomas Jefferson